Junk Food Diet Cookbook

Over 50 Comfort Food Recipes You Can Still Eat While on A Diet

by Olivia Rogers

Copyright © 2017 By Olivia Rogers
All rights reserved. No part of this book may be reproduced in any form without permission in writing from the author. No part of this publication may be reproduced or transmitted in any form or by any means, mechanic, electronic, photocopying, recording, by any storage or retrieval system, or transmitted by email without the permission in writing from the author and publisher.
For information regarding permissions write to author at Olivia@TheMenuAtHome.com
Reviewers may quote brief passages in review.

Please note that credit for the images used in this book go to the respective owners. You can view this at: TheMenuAtHome.com/image-list

Olivia Rogers
TheMenuAtHome.com

Table of Contents

Who is this book for? 6

What will this book teach you? 7

Introduction 8

Recipe 1: Healthy Whole Wheat and Oats Pumpkin Pancakes ... 10

Recipe 2: Low-Fat and Healthy Buttermilk Waffles 12

Recipe 3: Coconut Chocolate Energy Truffle Recipe 14

Recipe 4: Deep Dark Chocolate Layer Cake 16

Recipe 5: Low Fat Strawberry Cheesecake 18

Recipe 6: Creamy Cheese Chocolate Chip Cookies 21

Recipe 7: Low-Cal, Low-Fat Mashed Potatoes with Crispy Golden Chicken 23

Recipe 8: Crispy Golden Chicken 25

Recipe 9: Chicken Breasts Stuffed with Pimiento Cheese .. 27

Recipe 10: Black Bean and Quinoa Burgers 29

Recipe 11: Creamy Tarragon Chicken Salad 31

Recipe 12: Fish and Chips with Tartar Sauce 33

Recipe 13: Roasted Red Pepper, Hummus, Avocado & Feta Sandwich 35

Recipe 14: Mom's Easy Healthy Baked Beans 38

Recipe 15: Quick Fall Minestrone 40

Recipe 16: Healthier World's Best Lasagna 42

You can also add 43

Recipe 17: Low-Calorie Cauliflower Crust Pizza (Gluten Free) ... 44

Recipe 18: Spaghetti Squash and Tomato Casserole 46

Recipe 19: Mom's Creamy Chicken and Broccoli Casserole ... 48

Recipe 20: Ground Beef and Texas Bean Enchiladas _____ 50

Recipe 21: Low Salt, Low Fat Turkey Sloppy Joes _____ 52

Recipe 22: Sweet Potato Hash Browns _____ 54

Recipe 23: Curried Butternut Squash Bisque _____ 56

Recipe 24: Asparagus and Chicken Noodle Casserole _____ 58

Recipe 25: Harvest Port and Butternut Squash Stew _____ 60

Recipe 26: Halibut and Corn Chowder _____ 62

Recipe 27: Pork Kebabs with Honey _____ 64

Recipe 28: Four Bean Salad _____ 65

Recipe 29: Crock Pot Jambalaya _____ 66

Recipe 30: Sweet Potato Fish Cakes _____ 67

Recipe 31: Sweet Potato Fritters _____ 69

Recipe 32: Brown Sugar Barbecue Chicken _____ 70

Recipe 33: Chicken and Sweetcorn Macaroni _____ 72

Recipe 34: Confetti Spaghetti Salad _____ 74

Recipe 35: Beef and Curry Pasta _____ 75

Recipe 36: Tandoori Chicken _____ 77

Recipe 37: Spiced Salmon with Chili Sauce _____ 78

Recipe 38: Slow Cooked Stuffed Gammon _____ 79

Recipe 39: Potato and Pork Bake _____ 81

Recipe 40: Summer Cabbage Soup with Sausages _____ 82

Recipe 41: Teriyaki Fried Rice with Chicken _____ 83

Recipe 42: Sea Bass with Orange and Honey _____ 85

Recipe 43: Slow Cooker Breakfast Casserole _____ 86

Recipe 44: Slow Cooker Jambalaya _____ 88

Recipe 45: Spaghetti Bolognaise _____ 90

Recipe 46: Beef and Vegetable Parmesan _____ *92*
Recipe 47: Fried Green Tomatoes _____ *93*
Recipe 48: Mushroom and Cabbage Stroganoff _____ *95*
Recipe 49: Beef and Portobello Stroganoff _____ *96*
Recipe 50: Chili Con Carne _____ *98*
Recipe 51: Baked Sweet Potatoes with Sour Cream _____ *100*
Final Words _____ *101*
Disclaimer _____ *103*

Who is this book for?

This book will greatly benefit health conscious people who are also food lovers and yet want to stay fit and live a long life. Also, the recipes included in this book are for people who want or need to lose weight while still being able to have comfort foods.

A common-sense approach to healthy eating by focusing on what you can eat, and not on what you have to give up, will help you get results without feeling deprived. Once you know how many calories to consume, you can enjoy your meals with low calorie yet exceptionally tasty versions of your favorite foods, with the entire family.

What will this book teach you?

The key to accomplishing and continuing to remain healthy isn't about dietary changes on a short-term basis. It's about a way of life that comprises eating well, daily physical exercise, and balancing the number of calories you consume with the number of calories your body uses.

In this book, you can find:

- Great tasting recipes that are healthy too
- All recipes assessed by registered nutritionists
- Offers comfort foods that are satisfying for the whole family
- Dieting without having to give up some of your favorite foods
- Learn to eat sensibly and keep the weight off
- Low-calorie editions of hearty foods

Introduction

Dieting can be easier said than done for those that love food. A lot of people think dieting means eating only fruits and vegetables and the favorites they've come to love are not permissible at all. Now here is a cookbook that will guide you how to take pleasure in the foods you love, without feeling guilty.

Comfort foods in this cookbook offer the finest of both worlds. You'll get great tasting foods that are low in calories and will help in weight loss. All of the recipes are evaluated by dieticians and are the sort of foods that your whole family will relish. Home cooking presents a lot of options and full control over what you're eating. You would be amazed what little alterations can make some of your favorite foods healthier. Some of the recipes you will find are:

- Pizza
- Lasagna
- Strawberry Cheesecake
- Fried Chicken tenders
- Pumpkin Pancakes
- Mashed Potatoes
- Chocolate truffle.

Your dieting will not be successful if you aren't eating foods you get pleasure from. With this book, you can cook the kind of food you enjoy and view as comfort foods, but with a healthy twist on an old favorite for e.g. — if your recipe calls for deep-frying fish or chicken, try baking or grilling as these are healthier variations. Perhaps using lower-calorie ingredients for example if your lasagna recipe uses full-fat or whole milk, butter, and cheese, try making it with less butter, non-fat milk, light cream cheese, spinach and tomatoes-you might be amazed to find you have a new desirable dish! Just remember to keep your portion size normal.

Those of you with a sweet tooth can try out some new, exotic fruits and/or low-fat fruit yogurt, low fat ice-cream or use skim milk for your smoothies.

Recipe 1: Healthy Whole Wheat and Oats Pumpkin Pancakes

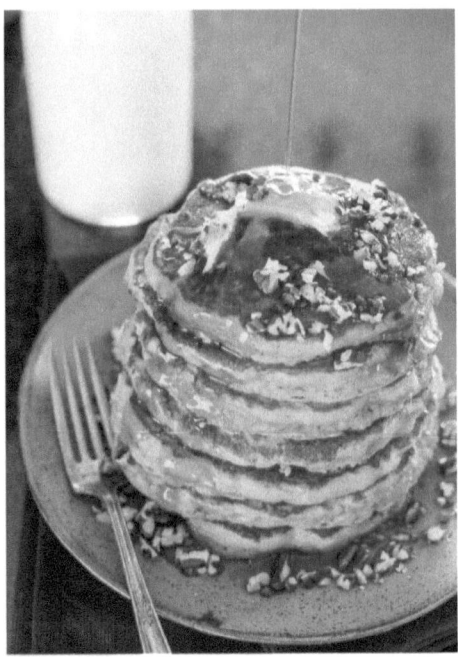

This healthy recipe for pancakes provides only 118 calories/81 grams. It is also a rich source of carbohydrates, fiber, proteins and a small amount of fat is also provided.

Buttermilk can be replaced by sour milk which can be easily made at home. Blend lemon juice or vinegar in 1 cup of nonfat milk. Set aside for 10 minutes before utilizing. For toppings roasted nuts can be used. Cook the nuts for 2 to 4 minutes in a small pan. The pan should be heated on medium flame. Stir till the nuts turn light brown.

Preparation time: 5 minutes
Total time: 5 minutes

Ingredients

- eggs (3 big)
- brown sugar (⅓ cup)
- apple sauce (½ cup)

- pumpkin puree (½ cup)
- buttermilk (1½ cup)
- vanilla extract (2 teaspoon)
- whole wheat flour (1 cup)
- rolled oats (1 cup)
- baking powder (2 tablespoon)
- salt (½ teaspoon)
- pumpkin spice (1 teaspoon)

Method

1. Mix the eggs, buttermilk, brown sugar, apple sauce and pumpkin puree together in a large bowl. The batter should be well combined. Then add the flour, vanilla, salt, pumpkin spice, baking powder and the oats. Mix again thoroughly to obtain a perfect batter.

2. Take a scooped spoon and half fill it with the prepared batter. Pour it in a pan heated on medium heat. Cook for 3 minutes so that the sides become firm then cook the other side of the pancake for about 1 to 2 minutes.

3. Sprinkle or spread maple syrup, butter or roasted pecans. To store these pancakes, keep in refrigerator in an airtight container.

Did You Know?

Fresh pumpkin puree contains just 50 calories and no fat, is a rich source of vitamin A, vital for vision and immunity. It also contains fiber and potassium, two very important nutrients.

Pumpkins remind us of Halloween, and those bred for jack-o-lanterns have a larger seed cavity, longer stems, and thinner walls for easier carving, while pumpkins for eating tend to be smaller and more solid. The flat white seeds that you scoop out are the unhulled, milder-tasting version of the smaller green seeds, or pepitas found in stores, Enjoy the white seeds as a snack, and add pepitas to salads, soups, or granola.

Recipe 2: Low-Fat and Healthy Buttermilk Waffles

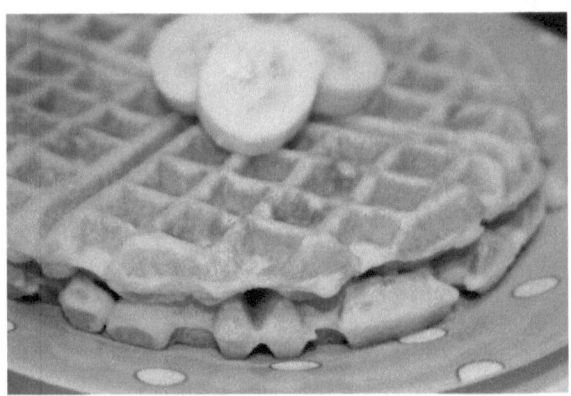

This waffle recipe is especially enjoyed by children and diet conscious people. It is easy to make and children also like making them. Each waffle only provides less than 100 calories, 3 g of fats and less than 15 g of carbohydrates.

Preparation time: 15 minutes
Cooking time: 10 minutes
Makes: 4 to 6 servings

Ingredients

- all-purpose flour (1 cup)
- toasted wheat germ (2 tablespoons)
- sugar (2 tablespoons)
- baking powder (1 teaspoon)
- baking soda (1/2 teaspoon)
- salt (1/4 teaspoon)
- nonfat or low-fat buttermilk (1 cup)
- vegetable oil (1 tablespoon)
- egg, lightly beaten (1 large)
- Cooking spray
- Maple syrup bananas (optional)

Method

1. In a measuring cup, mix flour, wheat germ, sugar, baking powder, baking soda and salt. In a separate bowl whisk oil, buttermilk and

egg together. Add this mixture to the dry one and whip until incorporated.

2. Preheat a waffle iron after applying the cooking spray. Pour quarter of a cup on the hot waffle, spreading it evenly. Let it cook for about 3 to 5 minutes or until the lights tell you. These waffles can be served with either bananas or maple syrup.

Note

This recipe will also work as pancakes. You may freeze leftover waffles by wrapping them tightly in foil and reheating them in a toaster oven.

Recipe 3: Coconut Chocolate Energy Truffle Recipe

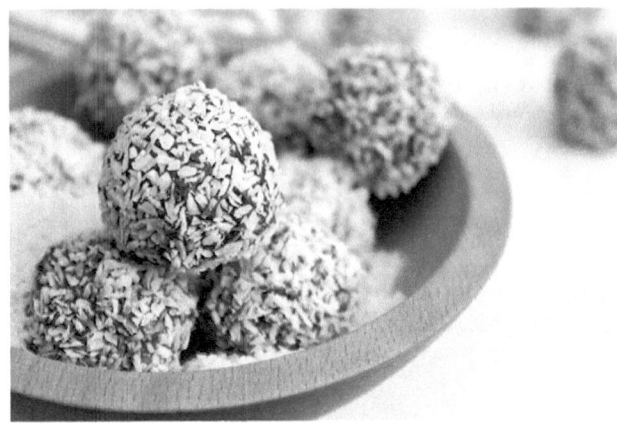

These creamy coconut-cocoa truffles, each one of them are fueled with revitalizing nutrients. These bite-sized snacks are powered by slow-burning natural sugars and protein. Have two truffles for your mid-afternoon snack, and you'll be fresh until dinnertime.

This recipe makes 40 truffles, with 92 calories per truffle, cooking time 45 minutes, total time 5-6 hours (including chill time)

Ingredients

For the truffles

- coarsely chopped, pitted medjool dates-2 cups
- boiling water-1 cup
- raw almonds-1 cup
- melted coconut oil-2 tablespoons
- vanilla extract-1 teaspoon
- sea salt-1/2 teaspoon
- coconut flour
- unsweetened cocoa powder 3/4 cup+3 tablespoons

For the chocolate coating

- dark chocolate cut into small pieces (8 ounces-70% cacao content or higher)
- coconut oil-2 tablespoons

- boiling water-1/2 cup
- unsweetened shredded coconut -1 cup

Method

1. Grind the almonds in a food processor until it turns into a creamy paste (for about 7 minutes). Add the dates and standing water, vanilla, coconut oil and salt to the processor. Blend until a smooth paste is formed, scraping down the sides a couple of times in between. Now put in the cocoa and coconut dough and process until a dough-like paste is formed. Refrigerate it for about 2-3 hours until very cold.

2. Line a baking tray with foil or parchment paper. Roll 40 balls out of the mixture using 1 tablespoon per truffle. Take coconut oil and chocolate in a heat-safe container. Add boiling water to it and mix gently with a spatula until the mixture becomes smooth.

3. With a fork dip each ball into the chocolate mixture and let the excess drip off. Prepare a separate tray of shredded coconut and roll the truffles to cover them fully. Transfer them to the prepared baking tray and refrigerate until the chocolate is set.

Did You Know?

Dates also known as nature's candy are a rich source of dietary fiber, iron and potassium. It is also a great source of B vitamins, which helps maintain energy levels. Almonds are one of the richest protein nuts, have satiating power and are high in monounsaturated fats and vitamin E.

Recipe 4: Deep Dark Chocolate Layer Cake

This deep dark chocolate layer cake makes 16 servings and provides 352 calories per slice. Also, it is low in fats and carbohydrates and contains almost no cholesterol. It is an ideal treat for people with a sweet tooth.

Ingredients

For the Cake

- Cooking spray
- all-purpose flour-3 cups
- Sugar-2 cups
- sifted natural unsweetened cocoa powder-2/3 cup
- baking soda-2 teaspoons
- teaspoon salt-3/4
- brewed coffee, at room temperature-1½cups
- canola oil-2/3 cup
- egg whites-2 large
- apple cider vinegar-2 tablespoons
- vanilla extract-2 teaspoons

For the Frosting

- egg whites-3 large
- sugar-1½cups
- cream of tartar-1/4 teaspoon

- Dash of salt
- vanilla extract-1 teaspoon

Method

1. Preheat oven to 350°F. Set a rack in the center of the oven; Apply cooking spray on 2 (9- x 1 1/2 -inch) round cake pans. Cover base of pans with parchment paper and spray with cooking oil; set it aside.

2. To prepare cake: Mix cocoa, flour, baking soda, sugar and salt in a big bowl, beating well. In another medium bowl, blend egg whites, vinegar, coffee, oil, and vanilla, mixing well. Incorporate coffee mixture into flour mixture, whisking until smooth. Separate batter uniformly between into the two ready pans; tap pan on a work surface to break air pockets.

3. Cook in the oven until a wooden toothpick placed in the center of the cakes comes out clean (around ½ hr. to 35 minutes.). Chill in pans on a wire rack for about 15-20 minutes. With a knife, loosen the edges of cakes by running it around the sides; turn cakes upside down onto a cooling frame. Take out the parchment; completely cool on rack.

4. To prepare frosting: Mix egg whites, cream of tartar, sugar and salt in a big deep heatproof bowl and set it over 1½inches of bubbling water; whip with an electric blender at medium-high speed (about 7 minutes). Remove bowl from saucepan; keep on beating until totally chilled (about 3 minutes). Blend in vanilla.

5. Carefully position 1 cake layer on a plate. Using a spatula spread a layer of frosting over it; now place the remaining cake. Evenly spread left over frosting over top and sides of complete cake.

Note

Unsweetened cocoa powder, egg whites and coffee, lightens up this fluffy favorite.

Recipe 5: Low Fat Strawberry Cheesecake

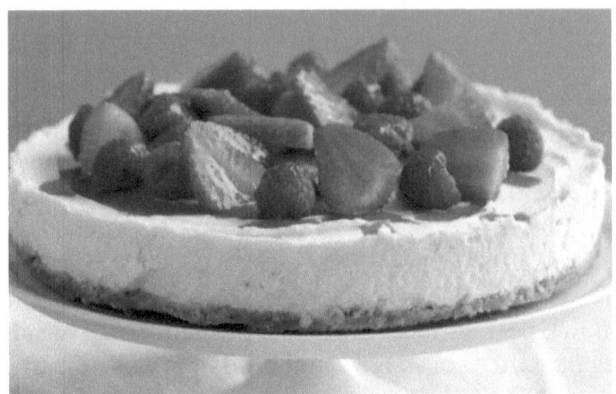

Serves: 8
Chill Time: 3 Hr
Cook Time: 35 Min

The next time someone tells you they're coming over, ask if they'd rather have a low-fat sweet dish or cheesecake. Of course, with this one you'll get the best of both slices after slice!

Ingredients

- 1% low-fat cottage cheese-16 ounces
- egg substitute*-3/4 cup
- reduced-fat cream cheese 4 ounces-softened
- sugar-1/3 cup+1 tablespoon (divided)
- vanilla extract-1 teaspoon
- low-fat vanilla yogurt-1/2 cup
- lemon juice-1/8 teaspoon
- sliced fresh strawberries-1 pint

Method

1. Preheat oven to 350°F. Coat a 9" pie plate with cooking spray. Combine cream cheese, cottage cheese, egg substitute, 1/3 cup sugar, and vanilla in a blender for 1 minute, until smooth. Pour into the prepared 9-inch pie plate. Bake for about half an hour to 40 minutes, or until the center is firm.

2. In a small bowl, combine remaining yogurt, 1 tablespoon sugar, and lemon juice and blend well. Spread uniformly over cheesecake, and then bake for 5 minutes. Take out from oven and cool entirely. Top with sliced strawberries, then cover loosely and chill for at least 3 hours prior to serving.

Note

Other toppings include a combination of blackberries, raspberries, and blueberries, or even sliced kiwifruit!

Read This FIRST - 100% FREE BONUS

FOR A LIMITED TIME ONLY – Get Olivia's best-selling book *"The #1 Cookbook: Over 170+ of the Most Popular Recipes Across 7 Different Cuisines!"* absolutely FREE!

Readers have absolutely loved this book because of the wide variety of recipes. It is highly recommended you check these recipes out and see what you can add to your home menu!

Once again, as a big thank-you for downloading this book, I'd like to offer it to you *100% FREE for a LIMITED TIME ONLY!*

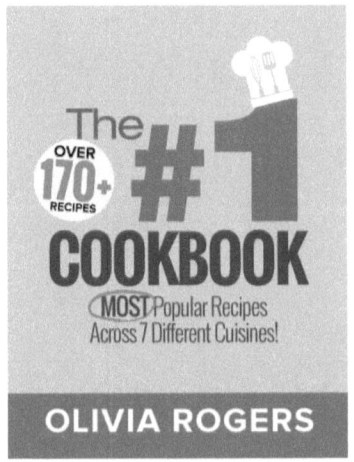

Get your free copy at:

TheMenuAtHome.com/Bonus

Recipe 6: Creamy Cheese Chocolate Chip Cookies

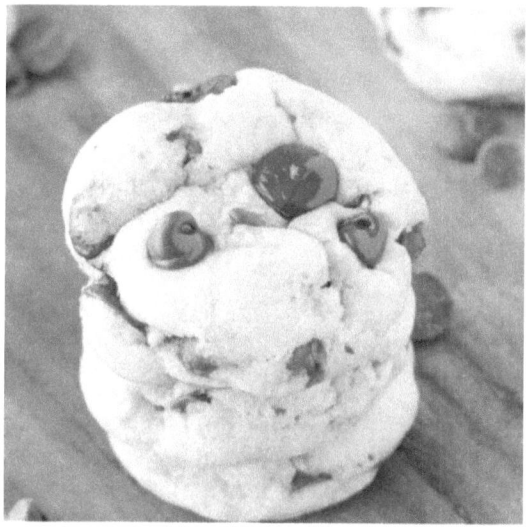

A holiday becomes a reason to eat more cookies and these tempting cheese cream cookies are some of the most delicious, lightest, softest, chewiest cookies ever to come out of the kitchen…Yet have just 40 calories… and less than 2 grams of fat each! Try and stop at just one.

(Makes about 10-12)

Ingredients

- 1/3 cup+1/4 cup oat flour OR
- Salt-1/8 tsp.
- Baking soda-1/4 tsp.
- dark chocolate chips 2-5 tbsp., or as desired
- sugar granules or xylitol 1/4 cup (46g)
- cream cheese(full-fat), such as Tofutti-3 tbsp. (45g)
- Pure vanilla extract-1/2 tsp.
- melted coconut oil-1 tbsp. (12g)

Method

1. In a deep bowl, combine the first 5 ingredients. In a cup, beat together the remaining 3 ingredients. If the cheese is too firm heat it a little so that it blends. Pour the wet ingredients into the dry,

then mix together and do not include extra liquid. Keep stirring and scraping off the spoon as you whip till it forms a smooth batter.

2. Shape into a big ball, then shape it into cookie dough balls and freeze for at least half an hour on a plate. Preheat oven to 325 F and grease a cookie tray, when ready to bake. Bake for 8 minutes—they will seem quite undercooked when they come out, wait for at least 10 minutes by which time they should harden.

Fun Fact

Cocoa and dark chocolate have many health benefits; they contain a large amount of antioxidants (flavonoids) which may assist in keeping high blood pressure down and lessen the risk of stroke and heart attacks. The darker the chocolate, the more beneficial it is. According to an Italian study, a small square (20g) of dark (bittersweet) chocolate every three days is the ideal dose for cardiovascular benefits. Eating more does not offer added benefits.

Recipe 7: Low-Cal, Low-Fat Mashed Potatoes with Crispy Golden Chicken

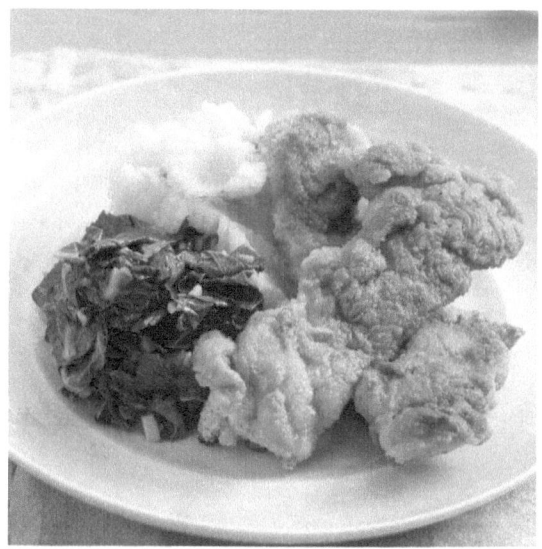

This is a low fat and low calorie (per 2/3-cup serving: 156 calories, 34g carbohydrate) version of the popular classic side dish.

To avoid an overload on carbohydrates, try adding cauliflower or some beans that are lower in carbs and have much higher protein content (and antioxidants) to give the consistency of classic mashed potatoes.

Yields: 6 servings
Preparation time: 20 minutes
Cooking time: 35 minutes

Ingredients

- garlic cloves 8 to 10
- quartered potatoes, 2 pounds (Yukon Gold recommended)
- light sour cream 1/3 cup
- fat-free milk 1/4 cup
- shredded fresh rosemary, oregano, or thyme-1 tablespoon
- salt 1/2 teaspoon
- black pepper 1/4 teaspoon

Method

1. To roast garlic, wrap unpeeled cloves in foil, bake at 400°F for about half an hour or until cloves feel squashy when pressed. Squeeze garlic from peels into a small bowl when cool enough.

2. Meanwhile, dip the potatoes in cold water a large saucepan and bring to a boil over high heat. Cook the potatoes on low heat or until tender, for about 20 minutes. Remove the potatoes and peel them.

3. With a potato masher or an electric mixer (on low speed), mash potatoes and garlic. Add milk, sour cream; herbs-oregano, rosemary, or thyme; salt; and black pepper. Whip until soft and fluffy.

Healthy Cooking Tips

The potatoes may become mushy if you directly place the potatoes in hot/warm water for boiling, the cold ingredients like milk and sour cream should be a room temperature before adding it to the hot potatoes. Do not over mix the ingredients.

The roasted garlic and the fresh herbs add a rich flavor to the potatoes, help in reducing cholesterol, and the low-fat sour cream gives a silky consistency and a dash of flavor.

Recipe 8: Crispy Golden Chicken

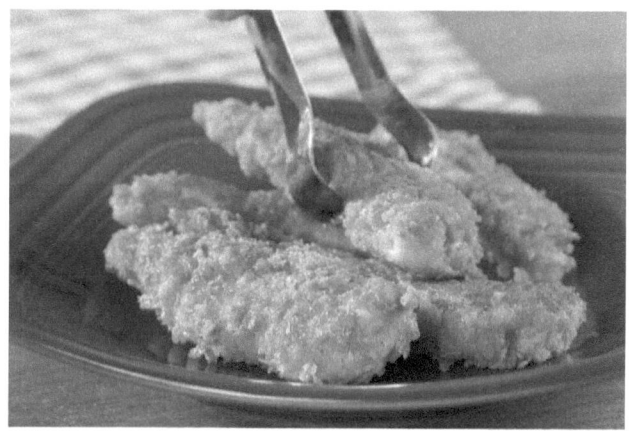

Chicken is a good source of protein, trim off the fat and prefer chicken breasts to legs or thighs as they contain less fat

Serves: 8
Preparation Time: 5 min
Cooking Time: 20 min

Ingredients

- 2 beaten egg whites,
- almond flour-1 cup (150 g)
- Paprika-1 tsp.
- Garlic powder-1 tsp.
- Salt-1/2 tsp.
- Black pepper-1/2 tsp.
- Dried thyme-1/2 tsp.
- chipotle powder-1 tsp. (optional)
- chicken breast tenders-2 pounds (900 g), rinsed and patted dry
- 2-4 tablespoon olive oil

Method

1. Whisk egg whites in a shallow dish. In another medium sized bowl, combine all dry ingredients, and mix well. Dip chicken in the beaten eggs mixture. And then cover it in the dry mixture.

2. In a medium sized skillet, heat oil and place the chicken in it and allow both sides to brown (about 3-4 minutes each side).

Cooking Tip

If you want crispier and very well-done chicken, place the fried pieces on a sheet pan in such a way that there is space between the pieces. Put chicken in oven for 10-15 minutes. Remove and serve.

Recipe 9: Chicken Breasts Stuffed with Pimiento Cheese

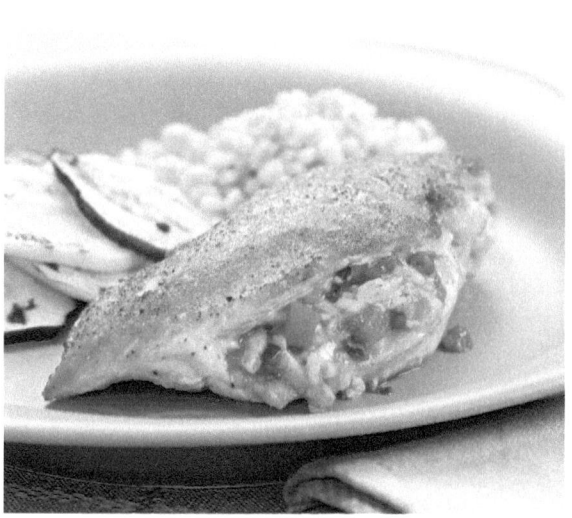

Filling skinless boneless, chicken breasts with scallions, pimientos and cheese gives them grand taste effortlessly. Don't be worried if some of the stuffing falls out while the chicken is baking; just scoop it up from the pan as you dish out. Serve with: Sautéed summer squash or zucchini and barley. It is an extremely nutritious dish with just 200 calories per serving, low in cholesterol, fats and carbohydrates. This recipe makes 4 servings and requires just 45 minutes in preparation.

Ingredients

- Gouda cheese, preferably smoked and shredded (1/2 cup)
- chopped scallion/green spring onions (2 tablespoons)
- sliced pimientos, chopped (1 tablespoon)
- paprika, divided (1 teaspoon)
- *chicken breasts 4 small boneless, skinless trimmed and tenders removed (total 1¼-1½ pounds)
- Salt (1/2 teaspoon divided)
- freshly ground pepper, divided (1/2 teaspoon)
- extra-virgin olive oil (1 tablespoon)

Method

1. Heat oven to 400 degrees. In a small bowl, mix pimientos, Gouda, scallion and ½ teaspoon paprika. Cut a slit in the side of the chicken length wise so that it opens like a book. Season the inside with salt and pepper.

2. Dividing the cheese equally among the breasts, press the block of cheese and close the chicken. Then rub the remaining salt, pepper and paprika on the outside of the chicken breasts.

3. Place the seasoned chicken in hot oil over medium heat. Cook for about 2 minutes until one side turns golden brown. Then flip the chicken on the other side, turn off the heat and place the cooking pan in the oven.

4. Let it bake until the chicken is not pink. To check if the chicken is well cooked insert an instant read thermometer in the inner of the chicken. If the thermometer reads 165 degrees or above, then your chicken is perfect.

Tips & Notes

If a small breast is not available, take off the tenders of a 5 to 6-ounce chicken breast. The tenders can be frozen and later be stir-fried.

You can add other ingredients to the stuffing inside the chicken for example mushrooms, broccoli and onions. It gives a unique taste and is more filling.

Recipe 10: Black Bean and Quinoa Burgers

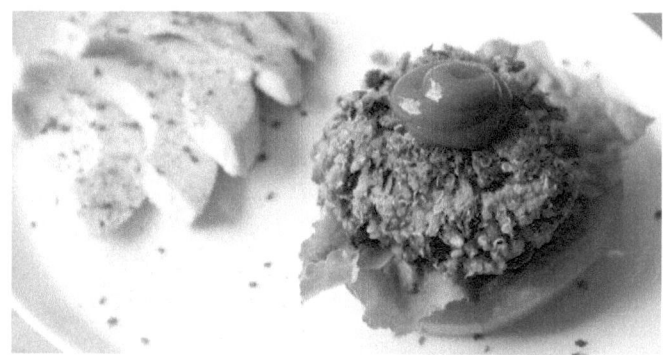

For more frequent burger urges, try something a tad healthier to overcome the craving. These black bean and quinoa burgers are packed with protein and fiber which leads to efficient digestion and a healthy heart. Toss these patties on a lettuce bun with avocado and a dollop of homemade ketchup, some chopped sliced tomato and it's a winning burger for both taste and nutrition! Place a slice of sharp cheddar if you're feeling indulgent.

Ingredients

- (15.5 ounces) black beans, rinsed and drained-1 can
- Cooked quinoa-1/2 cup
- Cumin- 1/2 teaspoon
- Freshly ground black pepper-1/2 teaspoon
- Paprika-1/2 teaspoon
- Sea salt1/2 teaspoon
- Nutritional yeast 1 tablespoon
- Extra-virgin olive oil (1 tablespoon) plus more for cooking

Method

1. Heat the oven to 400 degrees. Mash the beans in a bowl and mix well. The beans should be so well mashed that it is easy to shape into patties. Then make four equal patties. The ideal thickness for the patties is ¼ to ½ inch.

2. In an oven friendly dish heat ½ tablespoon olive oil on high heat and cook each side of patties in the oil for 1 minute or until light golden brown. Place the dish in the oven and cook for quarter of an

hour. After that remove dish from oven and enjoy with either fresh buns or green vegetables with any topping you desire.

Facts

Quinoa contains 8 grams/1 cup serving of protein when cooked. Quinoa is an excellent alternate for rice and *it's adaptable enough to make muffins, cookies, and breakfast dishes. It is packed with manganese, iron, fiber and magnesium. It is a unique plant based source of complete protein since it is totally gluten free.*

Recipe 11: Creamy Tarragon Chicken Salad

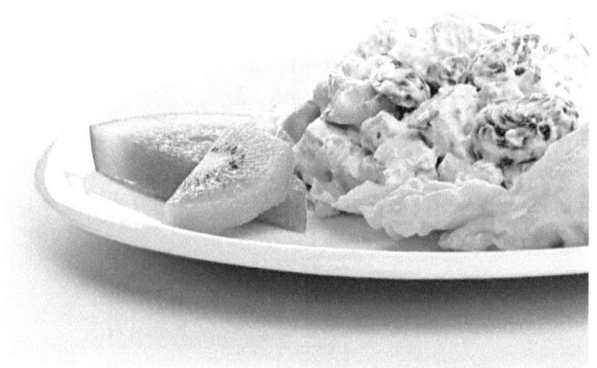

Ingredients

- boneless, skinless chicken breast, trimmed (2 pounds)
- reduced-sodium chicken broth (1 cup)
- walnuts, chopped (1/3 cup)
- reduced-fat sour cream (2/3 cup)
- low-fat mayonnaise (1/2 cup)
- dried tarragon (1 tablespoon)
- salt (1/2 teaspoon)
- freshly ground pepper (1/2 teaspoon)
- diced celery (1 1/2 cups)
- halved red seedless grapes (1 1/2 cups)

Method

1. Heat oven to about 450 degrees Fahrenheit. In a baking dish, place the chicken, making sure the chicken is evenly spread. Pour the broth and place in the oven for 30 to 35 minutes until the chicken center is not pinkish in color which can be checked by the instant read thermometer. After taking out the chicken from the oven, place it on the cutting board and leave it to cool down until it is cool enough to touch. Then dice it.

2. In the meantime, toast the walnuts in the oven, spread out on a baking tray, until fragrant and light golden. Then let them cool.

Mix mayonnaise, sour cream, salt, pepper and tarragon in a large container or bowl. Add in the walnuts, chicken and grapes and turn and mix to cover well.

Tips & Notes

You can make the chicken beforehand to save time. The chicken can be baked and refrigerated for up to 2 days. The salad can be kept chilled for up to a day and include the nuts just prior to serving.

Recipe 12: Fish and Chips with Tartar Sauce

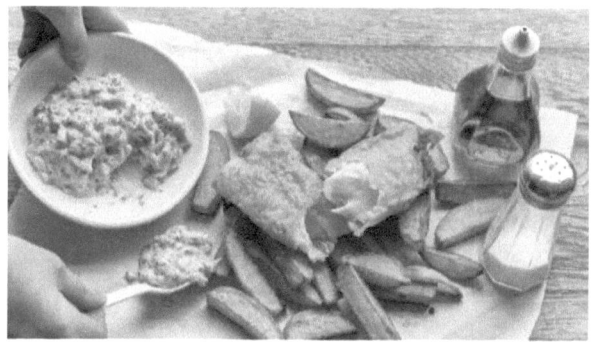

Servings: 4

Ingredients

For the Fish and Chips

- fat-free buttermilk-3/4cup
- fish fillets (catfish, tilapia, red snapper or your choice of firm fish fillets) 4(6 ounce)
- Potatoes, scrubbed and cut into sticks-1½lbs
- Paprika-3/4teaspoon
- salt-½teaspoon
- pepper-½teaspoon
- cornmeal-2/3cup
- Old Bay Seasoning-½teaspoon
- egg whites-2

For the Tartar Sauce

- fat-free mayonnaise-1/3cup
- scallion, chopped-1tablespoon
- unsweetened pickle, chopped-1tablespoon
- lemon juice-1teaspoon

Method

1. Add the fish into the buttermilk in a marinating dish or zip-lock bag, and mix well so that the fish is coated. Place the dish/bag in

the refrigerator and keep for at least half an hour or up to 2 hours, turning the fish occasionally. Keep oven ready at 425° F.

2. Cover with foil, two rimmed cookie sheets, inserting a rack in one of the pans. In the second pan, spray olive oil and spread potatoes evenly, sprinkle them with salt, paprika, and pepper; turn to coat.

3. Cook the potatoes in the oven for half an hour. On a sheet of wax paper or in a pie pan, blend together Old Bay Seasoning, the cornmeal and the remaining spices (1/4 tsp. each of paprika, salt and pepper) while the potatoes are baking.

4. In another bowl, whisk egg whites until frothy. Discard the buttermilk and take out the fish fillets. Coat both sides of the fish in egg whites, and then in the cornmeal mixture, shaking off excess.

5. Place the fish onto a clean sheet of wax paper or a plate. Spray olive oil on both sides of fish and then place fish evenly in the pan on top of the rack. Bake fish for about 15 minutes or until done golden brown. Simply combine the mayonnaise, pickle, scallion, and lemon juice, in a small bowl. While the fish and potatoes are cooking. Serve fish hot with tartar sauce and potatoes.

Recipe 13: Roasted Red Pepper, Hummus, Avocado & Feta Sandwich

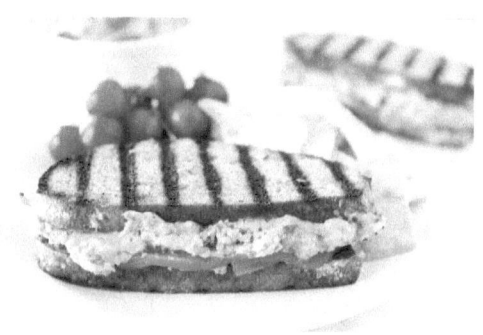

Makes: 2 sandwiches
Preparation Time: 5 minutes
Cooking Time: 10 minutes
Total Time: 15 minutes

This recipe is very flavorful and healthy. Its main ingredients are hummus, red pepper, feta cheese and avocado. The best part about this recipe is that it is less time consuming and easy to make.

Ingredients

- whole wheat bread (4 slices)
- hummus* (1/2 cup)
- ripe (pit less) avocados (2)
- crumbled feta cheese (1/4 cup)
- fresh lemon juice (2 teaspoons)
- freshly chopped basil (1 tablespoon)
- Salt and black pepper (to taste)
- roasted red peppers, drained (1/2 cup)

Method

1. Spread the hummus smoothly on the bread and keep aside. Using a fork mash the avocado and feta cheese in a bowl. Then mix in the basil and lemon juice. Season with salt and pepper.

2. Now spread this mixture over the bread with the hummus. Then add toasted red pepper and place the other slice of bread to make

the sandwich. Spread a bit of oil or butter on the outer sides of the bread and toast it in a pan for 2 to 3 minutes. It can also be enjoyed without toasting.

Tip

Along with red peppers thinly sliced kalamata olives, cucumbers and red onions can also be used.

Included here is the recipe of the Low-fat Hummus.

*Low-fat Spicy Hummus

This recipe of hummus provides 35.4 calories. It also provides sodium, proteins, fiber and good fats. It has no cholesterol and is low in carbohydrates.

Ingredients

- Low-sodium garbanzo beans, drained (15.5-ounce can)
- Fresh, squeezed lemon (1/2)
- Plain, fat-free yogurt (2 tablespoon)
- Fresh, peeled garlic (3-5 cloves)
- Salt (1/2 teaspoon)
- Water (1/4 cup)
- Cayenne Pepper (1 tablespoon)
- light olive oil (1 tablespoon)

Method

1. Heat the garlic in a microwave until they tenderize or for about 30 to 40 seconds. Wash the garbanzo beans and then add all the other items in the blender. Course until all is well combined.

2. The bean liquid can be used instead of olive oil to make the hummus less fatty. To reduce the amount of sodium you can exclude the salt and wash the beans thoroughly.

Recipe 14: Mom's Easy Healthy Baked Beans

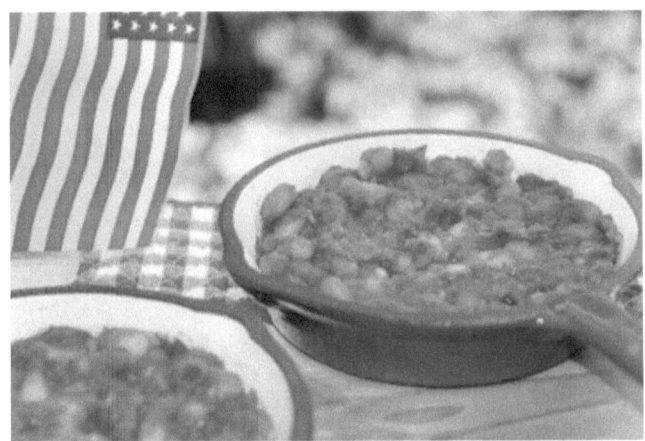

Mom's Healthy Baked Beans Secret Smokey Ingredient: This recipe's specialty is the liquid smoke which provides zero fats and a great taste to your food. The colgin or liquid smoke is a combination of vinegar, water, molasses, salt and a few other ingredients. Liquid smoke is also available in apple and pecan flavor

Serves: 8

Ingredients

- virgin olive oil (2 tablespoons)
- onions, finely chopped (2 cups)
- salt (to taste)
- organic tomato sauce (2 small cans)
- organic Worcestershire sauce (1 tablespoon + 1 teaspoon)
- liquid smoke (Hickory Flavor 4 tablespoons)
- mustard (¾ teaspoon)
- pure maple syrup (3 tablespoons)
- cannellini beans, rinsed and drained (2 cans)

Method

1. Heat oven to about 325°F. Sauté onions in heated oil over medium flame for 5 to 6 minutes. Sprinkle salt over it for taste.

2. Add the rest of the ingredients in the prepared onions and cook for another 5 minutes. Season to taste. Put the beans in a baking dish. Let the beans bake for 50 minutes.

Note

Beans are rich sources of protein, fiber and minerals. They are filling and will keep you satiated for long.

Even though molasses has high carbohydrate content, you need not worry about that since the other ingredients balance out its effect being low in carbohydrates.

Recipe 15: Quick Fall Minestrone

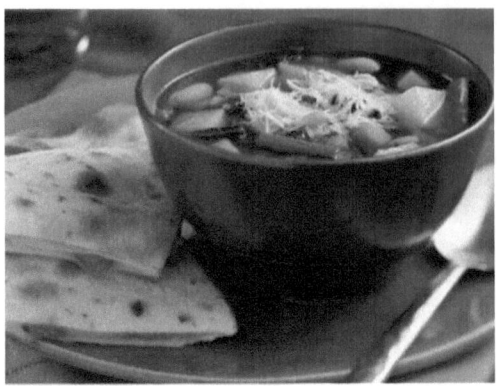

This recipe is a scrumptious meal made up of butternut squash and kale most enjoyed in the fall. This vegetarian soup is further made tastier and filling by adding beans and pasta.

Nutritional Information: This recipe provides proteins, fibers, sodium, calcium, iron and carbohydrates. It is also low in fats, cholesterol and provides only 212 calories.

Ingredients

- vegetable oil (1 tablespoon)
- chopped onion (1 cup)
- minced garlic (2 cloves)
- vegetable broth (6 cups)
- cubed peeled butternut squash (2 1/2 cups)
- cubed peeled baking potato (2 1/2 cups)
- cut green beans (1 cup)
- diced carrot (1/2 cup)
- dried oregano (1 teaspoon)
- freshly ground black pepper (1/2 teaspoon)
- salt (1/4 teaspoon)
- chopped kale (4 cups)
- uncooked orzo (1/2 cup)
- cannellini beans or other white beans, rinsed and drained (1 16-ounce can)
- grated fresh Parmesan cheese (1/2 cup)

Method

1. In a pan, heat oil and sauté the garlic and onion over medium heat for about 2 to 3 minutes until it softens. Then add the other ingredients except for kale, orzo, beans and cheese into the pan and cook until it comes to a boil.

2. Then lower the flames and keep stirring for 3 minutes. Then mix in the beans, kale and orzo and cook for a further 5 minutes. Top the grated cheese over it.

Recipe 16: Healthier World's Best Lasagna

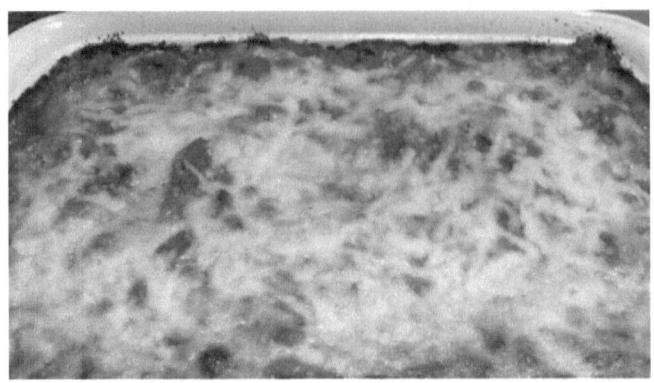

This low calorie and scrumptious recipe is really wholesome and healthy. It is another way for diet conscious people to enjoy their favorite meals. It is also a high protein recipe. To make it low fat, the parmesan cheese and salt have been left out.

Ingredients

- lean ground turkey-1½ pound
- minced onion-1/2 cup
- crushed garlic, 4 cloves
- 1 can crushed tomatoes-(28 ounce)
- tomato paste-1can (6 ounce)
- Water-1/2 cup
- dried basil leaves-1 teaspoon
- fennel seeds-1/2 teaspoon
- Italian seasoning-1 teaspoon
- ground black pepper-1/4 teaspoon
- chopped fresh parsley-2 tablespoons
- lasagna noodles-8
- 1 (8 ounce) fat-free ricotta cheese
- 1 (6 ounce) package shredded part-skim mozzarella cheese, divided

Method

1. Heat a large frying pan or Dutch oven over medium heat; cook for about 15 minutes and stir, ground turkey, garlic and onion, until

well browned. Blend in tomato paste, crushed tomatoes, and water. Season with Italian seasoning, basil, fennel seeds, pepper, and 2 tablespoons parsley. Simmer for about 1½ hours, uncovered, stirring occasionally.

2. Keep oven ready at 375°F (190°C). Bring to boil a large pot of lightly salted water. Cook lasagna in the boiling water, stirring seldom until cooked but stiff to bite, for about 8 minutes. Drain out the water.

3. Spread 1½ cups turkey sauce in the bottom of a baking dish. Arrange 4 noodles lengthwise over sauce. Spread the ricotta over noodles. Top with half of the mozzarella cheese. Spoon 1½ cups turkey sauce over mozzarella. Envelop with aluminum foil; make certain foil does not come in contact with the cheese to avoid sticking.

4. Bake in preheated oven until sauce is hot and cheese has melted, about 25 minutes more. Remove foil and bake until cheese is golden brown, about 25 minutes. Cool for 15 minutes before serving.

Cooking Tip

You can also add butternut squash, fresh spinach, or zucchini for added flavor.

Recipe 17: Low-Calorie Cauliflower Crust Pizza (Gluten Free)

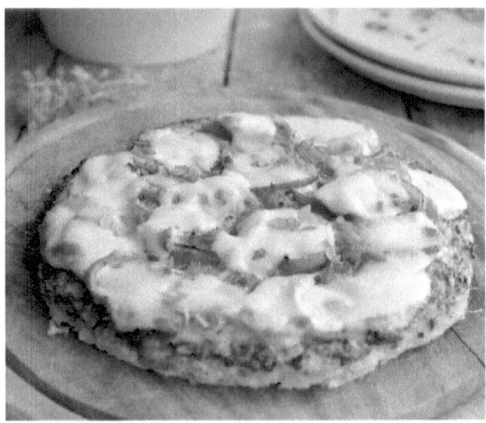

This pizza recipe is far healthier than the restaurant pizzas and is also appetizing. It comprises of a delicious wheat, tortilla and cauliflower crust topped with yummy vegetables and cheese. Be creative and make a flavorful pizza. It also provides a good amount of proteins and fiber which is very useful for the proper functioning of the heart.

Ingredients

- raw cauliflower, fresh or frozen (340g)
- egg (1 large)
- low-fat mozzarella cheese, grate 50g and slice the remaining 25g for the topping (75g)
- finely grated Parmesan cheese (2 tablespoons)
- dried basil (1/4 teaspoon)
- dried oregano (1/4 teaspoon)
- garlic granules or powder (1/4 teaspoon)
- salt (to taste)
- fresh black pepper (to taste)
- fresh tomatoes, thinly sliced (2)
- red onion, peeled and thinly sliced (1/2)
- fresh garlic, peeled and minced (2 cloves)
- red chili flakes (1/4 teaspoon)
- fresh oregano or basil (to garnish)

Method

1. Line a pizza tray with parchment paper. Heat oven to 210 degrees. Grate the cauliflower or process in a blender to obtain fine crumbs. But take care not to make it in a puree.

2. To soften the cauliflower crumbs, microwave it for at least 5 to 6 minutes. Add the egg, parmesan cheese, salt, cauliflower crumbs, mozzarella cheese, herbs, garlic powder and pepper in a bowl. Mix thoroughly until incorporated.

3. Flatten the dough in a 12.5cm large circle with 1.5cm thickness. Brush oil over it and bake it in the oven for 15 to 20 minutes or until golden brown. Then top the pizza crust with tomatoes, chili flakes, onion and garlic. Then cover it all with the cheese.

4. Keep the pizza in the oven and let it bake for 10 minutes until the cheese has completely melted and the topping are cooked well. Sprinkle oregano or basil as seasoning.

Note

This pizza recipe is a low calorie one and suitable for people on Paleo diet and is also a vegan recipe. Each slice contains 240 calories and is very filling and tasty to eat.

Recipe 18: Spaghetti Squash and Tomato Casserole

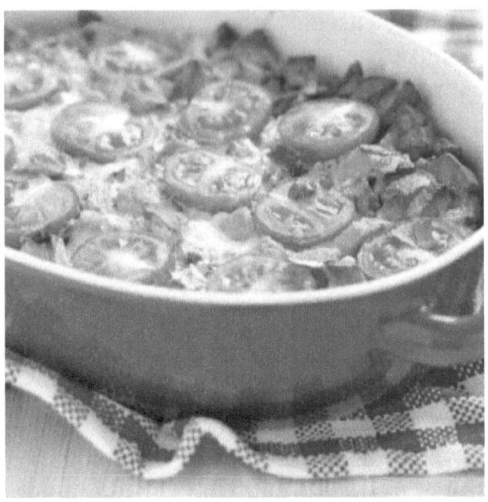

Few things are more calming than an enormous bowl of pasta with marinara sauce. But that means a lot of carbs? This "pasta" casserole substitutes the classic pasta with waistline-friendly spaghetti squash to fill those cravings without the extra calories and carbs. For the perfect healthy comfort food dinner, serve with a salad.

Ingredients

- spaghetti squash-1
- large carrots, diced-2
- large yellow onion, diced-1
- (28oz) crushed tomatoes-1 large can
- basil (dried or fresh)-1 teaspoon
- dried oregano-½ teaspoon
- garlic, chopped-3 cloves
- low-fat or part-skim mozzarella, grated-¼ pound
- extra-virgin olive oil-2 tablespoons
- grated Parmesan cheese-½ cup (optional)

Method

1. Slice squash laterally and put it in a baking dish filled with 1 inch of water making the skin face down. Preheat the oven at 350

degrees and cover the dish with a foil and cook for about 45 minutes, making sure the squash is tender.

2. In the meantime, sauté the carrots and onion in hot olive oil for 10 minutes. Then sprinkle salt and pepper for flavor. Cook basil, oregano, garlic, crushed tomatoes and the prepared vegetables in an open vessel for quarter of an hour.

3. While the sauce is cooking take out the squash from the oven and let it cool enough so that it can be easily handled. Take out the seeds. Using a fork scrape the flesh. If the flesh comes off like spaghetti, then you squash is well baked.

4. Now add the squash to the sauce that was cooking and turn off the stove mix all ingredients together. Then start layering the squash mixture and cheese alternately. First add squash mixture and then cheese and keep doing this until 8he sauce has finished.

5. Place the dish in the oven for at least half an hour, making sure the cheese is well melted. Set aside for about 15 to 20 minutes to let it cool and set completely.

Note

The flesh of spaghetti squash comes out in long threads, very much akin to the noodles for which it is called. In this recipe, the 'noodles' are thrown with vegetables and feta cheese. You can use a variety of vegetables, but be certain to use ones that have contrasting colors."

Grating the mozzarella cheese would be easier if it is frozen for 10 to 20 minutes.

Recipe 19: Mom's Creamy Chicken and Broccoli Casserole

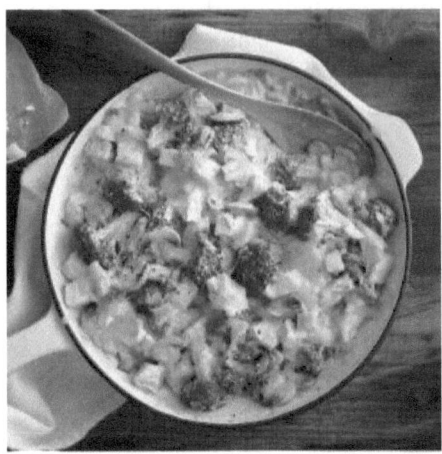

This recipe of creamy chicken provides less calories compared to the traditional one. It is lighter and also a yummy way of staying healthy and fit.

Nutritional Information: This dish provides only 277 calories and is also a great source of proteins, carbohydrates and fiber. It provides sodium, calcium and iron. It is low in fats and cholesterol.

Ingredients

- Steam-in-bag broccoli florets (1 12-ounce package)
- Canola oil (1 tablespoon)
- Already chopped onion (1 cup)
- pre-sliced mushrooms (2 8-ounce packages)
- all-purpose flour (3 tablespoons)
- fat-free milk (1 1/2 cups)
- chopped skinless, boneless rotisserie chicken breast (about 3 cups)
- plain fat-free Greek yogurt (1/2 cup)
- canola mayonnaise (1/4 cup)
- freshly ground black pepper (1/2 teaspoon)
- salt (1/4 teaspoon)
- sharp cheddar cheese, shredded (about 1/2 cup)
- Parmesan cheese, grated (about 1/4 cup)

Method

1. Heat the broiler. Microwave broccoli according to the instruction given on the package. Heat oil in a skillet on medium heat. Spread the oil and then put in the onions and mushrooms. Cook for about 10 to 12 minutes until the mushrooms turn brown, taking care not to burn it.

2. Then sprinkle flour over the prepared mixture and keep stirring for a minute. Then add the milk and stir until it boils. Cook for 3 minutes until it becomes of a thicker consistency.

3. Put in the chicken and broccoli and cook for a further 1 minute. Then turn off the heat and mix in the salt, pepper, yoghurt and mayonnaise. Evenly spread the cheese and then let it broil for about 2 to 3 minutes.

Recipe 20: Ground Beef and Texas Bean Enchiladas

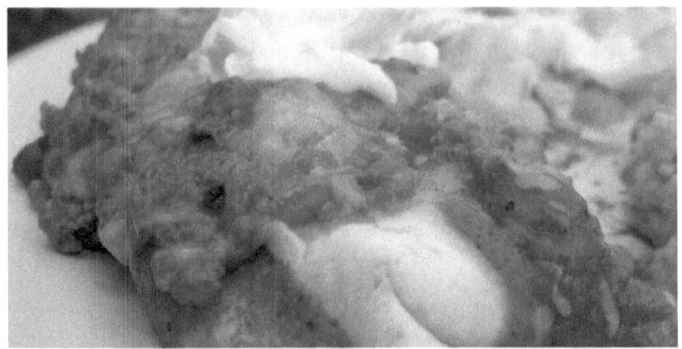

This recipe is a remake of the traditional one. It is easy to make and is simple.

Preparation time: 20 minutes
Cooking time: 20 minutes
Total time: 40 minutes

Ingredients

- ground beef (1 pound)
- pinto beans or black beans or Texas ranch style
- beans (1 15 ounces can)
- drained diced tomatoes (1 14 ounces can)
- finely diced fresh poblano peppers (1/2cup) or diced green chilies (1 4 ounces can)
- finely diced white onions (1/2cup)
- crushed garlic (2cloves)
- shredded Mexican blend cheese or Monterey Jack Cheese (1cup)
- salt and pepper (to taste)
- (12 -15 8-inch) flour tortillas or whole wheat
- flour tortillas or corn tortillas

Enchilada Sauce

- hot water (2 1/4cups)
- tomato paste (1 6 ounces can)
- margarine or butter (2tablespoons)
- flour (2tablespoons)

- red chili powder (5 teaspoons)
- cumin (1 teaspoon)
- garlic powder (2 teaspoons)
- salt and pepper (to taste)

Method

1. Heat oven to 350 degrees. In a skillet mix onion, garlic, salt, pepper and ground beef. Cook until beef turns brown. Then let the grease drain. Then put in the canned chilies, peppers, beans of your choice and tomatoes in the skillet.

2. Lower the heat, cover the dish and stir occasionally. In the meanwhile, prepare the sauce. Add all the ingredients required to make the sauce in a bowl and whip until all is completely combined. Then sprinkle the salt and pepper.

3. Transfer ½ cup of sauce in the prepared meat mix. Then quickly turn off the heat. Coat each tortilla in the prepared sauce making sure it is completely covered.

4. In a pan place the sauce covered tortillas. Then put the meat mixture on one side of it and roll it. After rolling make sure that the open side is on the bottom so that the contents do not spill.

5. Any remaining mixtures can be spread over the enchiladas. Wrap in foil and let it bake for 15 minutes. After removing the enchiladas from the oven, open the foil and evenly top with grated cheese. Put it in the oven again for 5 minutes so that the cheese melts. Cut the enchiladas into half and serve with either guacamole or rice or sour cream.

Recipe 21: Low Salt, Low Fat Turkey Sloppy Joes

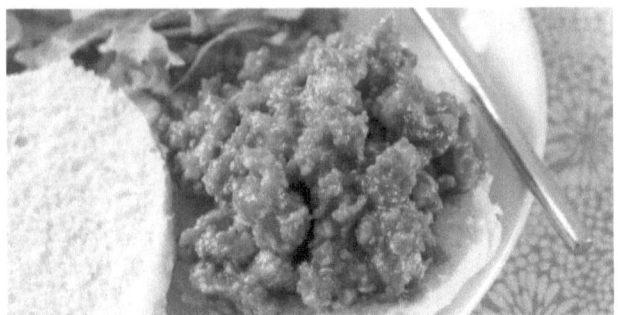

Servings: 6
Makes: 4 Sandwiches

Ingredients

- lean ground turkey (1 pound)
- onion (2/3 cup)
- green pepper (1/2 cup)
- jalapeno peppers (2)
- no-salt-added ketchup (1 cup)
- brown sugar (2 tablespoons)
- Worcestershire sauce (2 tablespoons)
- garlic powder (1 tablespoon)
- chili powder (2 tablespoons)
- mustard powder (1 tablespoon)
- salt (1/4 teaspoon)
- extra virgin olive oil (2 tablespoons)

Method

1. Dice the jalapenos after removing the seeds inside it. Also chop the onions and green pepper finely. Sauté the chopped items in a pan and keep aside. Then cook the turkey and drain it.

2. In a pan over medium heat stir in all the ingredients for 3 to 5 minutes. Lower the heat and let it simmer for 8-10 minutes so that the flavors blend well. You can serve it on crusty rolls or any kind of bread you prefer.

Cooking tips

If you do not want it too hot, cut down the jalapenos or add more according to taste.

Also, you may reduce the amount of brown sugar and try adding diced tomatoes and olives if you wish.

Recipe 22: Sweet Potato Hash Browns

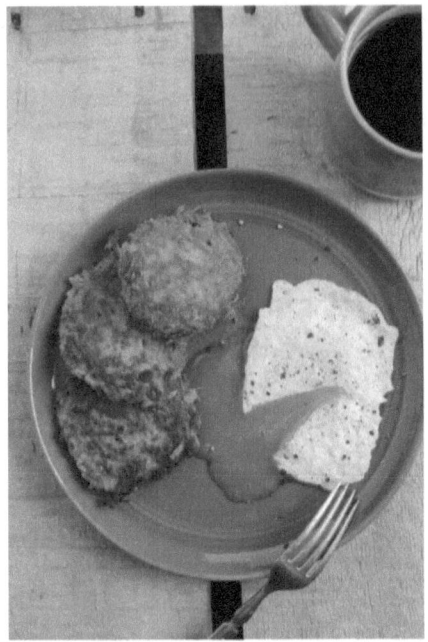

A traditional American comfort food to lift you out of any bad mood and warm you up completely

Serves 2

Ingredients

- 1 pound diced sweet potatoes
- 3 tablespoon virgin olive oil
- 1 small onion, chopped
- 1 tablespoon chopped fresh parsley
- Salt and ground pepper

Method

1. Boil potatoes in salted water until tender but still firm to the touch. Rinse under cold water before chilling thoroughly. Heat 1 tablespoon oil in a pan over medium heat and sauté onions until soft and browned then set aside.

2. Add remaining oil to pan and add potatoes and stir as they cook until slightly browned. Add onions and allow to cook for a minute before tossing in parsley. Add seasoning and serve.

Did You Know?

Allowing the potatoes to chill after they are boiled averts disintegration when they are sautéed.

Recipe 23: Curried Butternut Squash Bisque

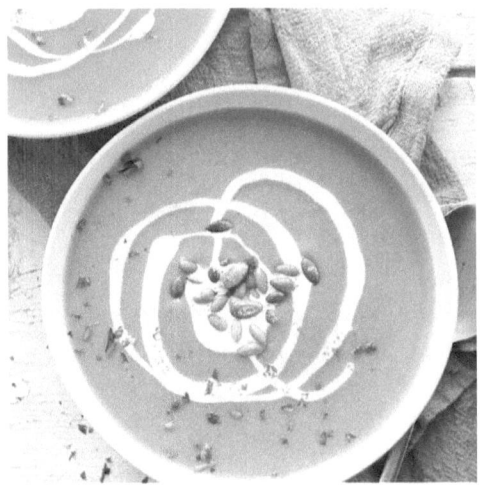

This creamy non-dairy soup allows you to eat clean and is a comforting meal that you can make in the comfort of your home. Great taste with no guilt attached.

Ingredients

- 1 teaspoon vegetable oil
- 1 chopped onion
- 2 minced cloves of garlic
- 3 cups peeled and chunked butternut
- 2 teaspoons curry paste
- 2 ½ cups water
- ½ cup coconut milk
- Salt to taste

Method

1. Heat oil over medium heat and sauté onion and garlic for twelve minutes. Add curry paste and sauté for a minute more. Add water and the butternut and allow to boil before reducing the heat. Cover pot and simmer until butternut is soft.

2. Place mixture in blender and blend until smooth. Pour in the coconut milk then blend it in until mixture looks creamy. Put back

into original pot and add seasoning as you reheat until steamy. Serve hot.

Note

This soup is so delicious that it carries the danger of preventing other parts of the meal being eaten after your family or guests fill up on it.

Recipe 24: Asparagus and Chicken Noodle Casserole

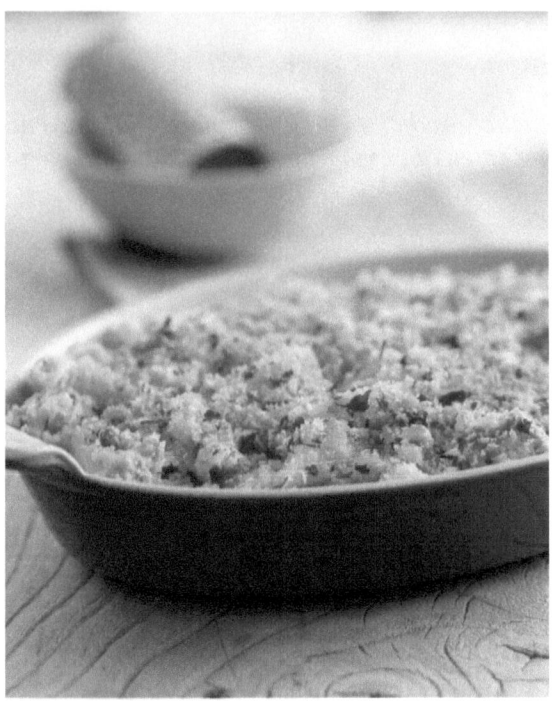

This comforting meal will give you a change from the usual and it is so flavorful that it will turn you into a fan for life.

Ingredients

- 2 bunch trimmed asparagus
- 8 ounces dry and wide noodles of choice
- 2 minced cloves of garlic
- 2 tablespoons each of flour, virgin olive oil and butter
- ½ cup chopped onions
- 1 cup cream of mushroom soup
- 3 cups milk
- Salt and pepper to taste
- Flesh of a whole chicken, cooked and cubed
- 6 ounces grated cheddar cheese
- ½ cup bread crumbs

Method

1. Place the asparagus in a pot of boiled and salted water and cook for a minute. Remove and rinse in cold water then set aside. Use same water to cook noodles following package instructions, less a minute cooking time, drain and stand.

2. Preheat oven to 175 degrees C. Sauté onions for 3 minutes over low heat in melted butter. Stir in flour and garlic and cook for a further 2 minutes, stirring. Add in the mushroom soup, milk and seasoning and continue to stir briskly until it thickens. Remove from heat and add to the noodles. Add chicken, half the cheese and asparagus and combine thoroughly.

3. Place mixture into an oven-proof dish and sprinkle the remaining cheese on top. Thoroughly mix together the olive oil and bread crumbs and spread mixture over casserole. Bake for 30 minutes until nicely browned.

Did You Know?

There is a museum in Germany, solely dedicated to asparagus. You get info about its history, how it is cultivated and many other aspects of this vegetable, dubbed 'The food of the gods' by one of the ancient Egyptian queens.

Recipe 25: Harvest Port and Butternut Squash Stew

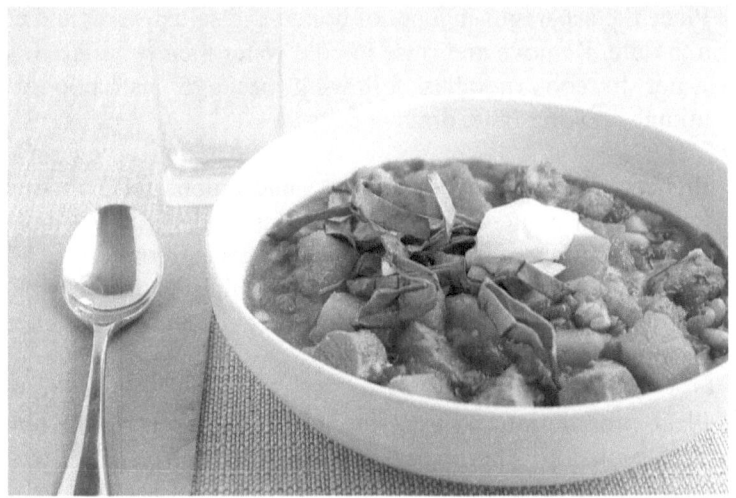

If you want a home cooked meal of restaurant quality, taste and flavor; this is it. You get the best of both worlds in one.

Ingredients

- 3 tablespoons flour
- 1 tablespoon each of olive oil and paprika
- 1 teaspoon each of ground coriander and salt
- pound boneless pork shoulder, cubed
- 2 cups each of chicken broth and peeled and cubed butternut
- 1 cup each of undrained diced tomatoes and thawed frozen corn
- 1 can baby lima beans
- 1 chopped onion
- 2 tablespoons vinegar
- 1 bay leaf

Method

1. Mix thoroughly 2 tablespoons of the flour, coriander, paprika and salt. Thoroughly coat pork and shake off access. Heat oil in a large thick base saucepan and brown the pork a little at a time. Place into crock pot and add all ingredients except flour, beans and broth.

2. Separately combine flour and broth and mix until smooth. Stir into the crock pot and cook covered over low heat for 9 hours. Add the baby lima beans 30 minutes before end of cooking time. Remove from pot and discard bay leaf before serving.

Note

You can substitute the baby lima beans for edamame of frozen cut green beans and the stew would still taste good.

Recipe 26: Halibut and Corn Chowder

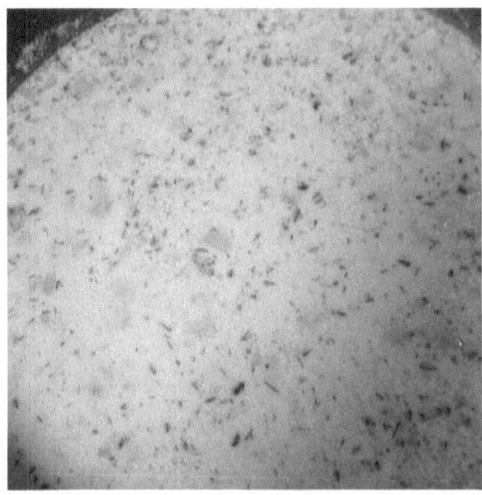

This is a versatile soup you can use with many dishes. You can use any firm fish in place of halibut and you can also experiment with different spices and seasoning.

Ingredients

- 1 red potato, cubed
- ½ large onion, chopped
- ½ cup each of milk and chopped celery
- 1x8 ounces can low sodium chicken broth
- ½ minced garlic clove
- ½ teaspoon salt
- ¼ teaspoon dried marjoram
- 1 tablespoon each of flour and butter
- 1 can each of cream-style corn & drained de-boned & flaked halibut
- 1 cup heavy cream

Method

1. Mix potatoes, celery, onion, garlic, chicken broth, marjoram and salt on a saucepan. Bring to boil over medium heat, reduce heat and simmer for 10 minutes. Whisk in the cream, milk.

2. Mix corn and flour then stir mixture into soup. Heat until slightly thickened, do not allow mixture to boil. Add the fish and stir gently to avoid flaking. Allow to heat through before serving

Fast tip

This soup is rather pale and leaving the skin on the potatoes will give it a bit of color.

Recipe 27: Pork Kebabs with Honey

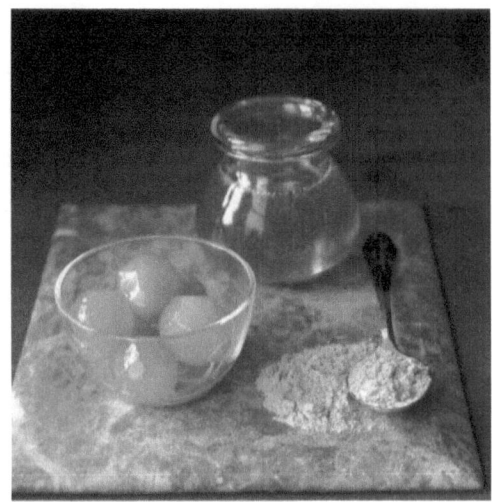

Pork is high in protein, making it filling and able to keep hunger away for longer. The dish therefore offers you comfort without making you feel guilty about it.

Ingredients

- 1½ pounds pork rashers without rind
- 6 peeled and halved baby onions
- 1 tablespoon mustard
- 3 tablespoons honey

Method

1. Preheat oven to 200 °C. Thread the meat onto kebab skewers alternating with the onions.

2. Mix honey and mustard and use mixture to brush kebabs. Arrange on oven rack and bake for 12-15 minutes.

Did you know?

Pope John Paul XXII loved mustard so much that he created a new Vatican position of mustard-maker to the pope in the early 1300s.

Recipe 28: Four Bean Salad

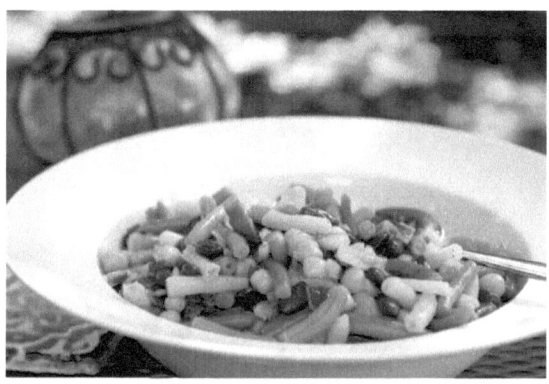

This salad tastes great and is a great source of energy. It will ensure that you do not get hunger pangs every now and again. In addition, beans are very nutritious and are a high-level protein food.

Ingredients

- 1 ½ cups blanched green beans
- 1 cups cooked speckled red beans
- 1 1/4 cups cooked white beans
- 1 each of green peppers medium onions, sliced
- ½ cup each white vinegar and olive oil
- 1 ½ tablespoons caster sugar
- ¼ cup chopped fresh coriander
- Salt and pepper

Method

1. Mix beans, peppers and onions in a salad bowl. Place remaining ingredients into a jug and whisk to make the salad dressing. Drizzle salad dressing over salad and immediately serve.

Olives Fun Fact

The olive tree lives for hundreds of years and olives are harvested for the first time after a tree is 15 years old. Fresh oil tastes better and is better used for salads and after a year it is better used for cooking.

Recipe 29: Crock Pot Jambalaya

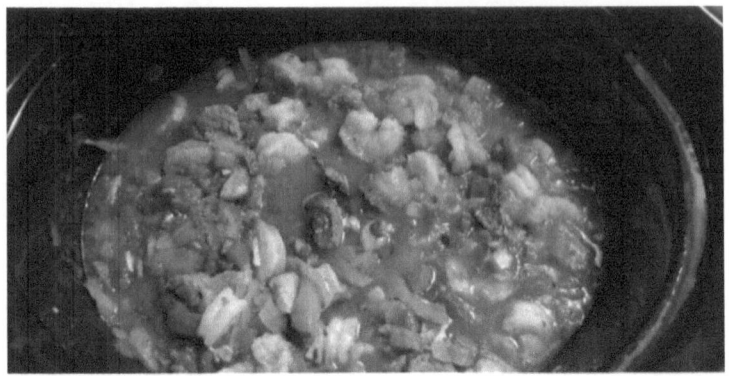

Jambalaya is a favorite in many American households and likely to bring back the memories of the good old days.

Ingredients

- 1 cup chopped onion
- 1 cup chopped green pepper
- 1 cup chopped celery
- 2 garlic cloves, minced
- 1 28 ounces can un-drained diced tomatoes
- ¾ pound cooked prawns
- 2 cups turkey sausage or smoked sausage
- ¼ teaspoon each of hot sauce and pepper
- ½ teaspoon each of salt and dried thyme
- 1 tablespoon dried parsley

Method

1. Add all ingredients except prawns and stir well. Cook on high for 3-4 hours. Add prawns to crock pot for the last 15 minutes of cooking time.

Note

There are variant types of prawns and you can easily substitute one for the other though they may slightly differ in flavor and taste.

Recipe 30: Sweet Potato Fish Cakes

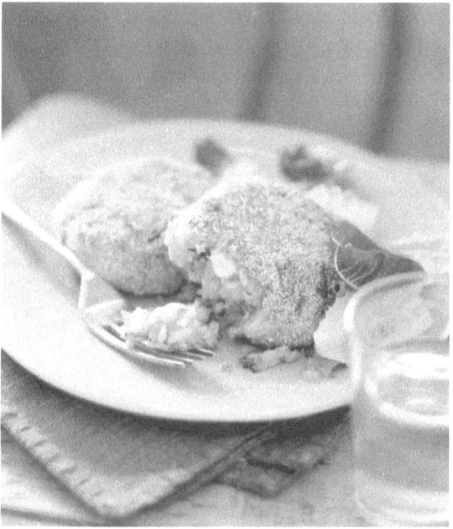

Fish cakes are nutritious and give you the desired comfort and they are a healthy snack that gives you no guilt feelings.

Ingredients

- 1-pound hake or whiting steaks
- 2 sweet potatoes, cooked and mashed
- 1 onion, grated
- 3 tablespoons chopped parsley
- 2 teaspoons lemon juice
- 2 beaten eggs
- 4 tablespoons coconut flour
- Salt and pepper

Method

1. Grease your crock pot. Put fish into blender and blend slightly. Mix fish with rest of ingredients. Shape mixture into six cakes. Sprinkle flour on a board and roll the fish cakes.

2. Place individually in crock pot. Close and cook on medium for four hours. Put in oven and grill for 2 minutes before serving.

Did you know?

Eggs contain proteins, folic acid and vitamin D. These increase alertness, a lack of vitamin D is associated with depression and reduced mental function

Recipe 31: Sweet Potato Fritters

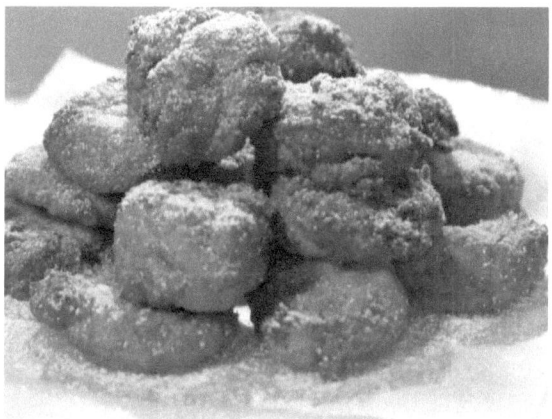

Sweet potato snacks will keep you full for longer and therefore help you eat less and, the sweet variety of potatoes is the healthier cousin.

Ingredients

- 1 pound grated sweet potatoes
- 10 ounces chopped onions
- ½ cup almond flour
- 1 beaten egg
- 1 teaspoon mixed spice
- Salt and pepper
- 2 tablespoon coconut oil

Method

1. Thoroughly mix all ingredients except oil in a bowl. Heat oil in pan and spoon mixture into pan to make several fritters.

2. Slightly press spooned mixture. Fry until crispy and browned then turn and repeat.

Did you know?

Sweet potatoes are versatile vegetables which you can enjoy boiled, fried, roasted, baked, pureed, steamed or grilled.

Recipe 32: Brown Sugar Barbecue Chicken

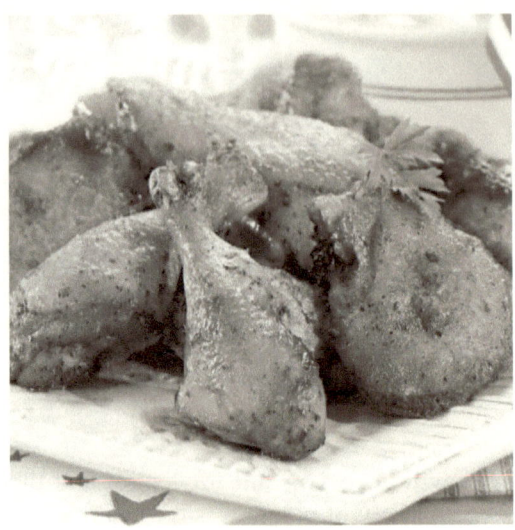

Even the pickiest of eaters are likely to be taken in by this simple and sweet sauce. You will get all the comfort and it really is finger licking good.

Ingredients

- 2 cups tomato sauce
- 1 cup brown sugar
- 2 tablespoons each of Worcestershire sauce and vinegar
- Salt and pepper
- 6 pounds chicken drumettes

Method

1. Preheat oven to 220 degrees C. Whisk together all ingredients except chicken. Use aluminum foil to line 2 baking trays. Toss chicken with one cup sauce then divide them into the two baking trays.

2. Bake on top shelves for 35 minutes, turning them after 15 minutes. When done, toss with ½ cup sauce and use remaining sauce for serving

Did You Know?

Drumettes are the thickest part of a chicken wing, which resembles a small drumstick.

Recipe 33: Chicken and Sweetcorn Macaroni

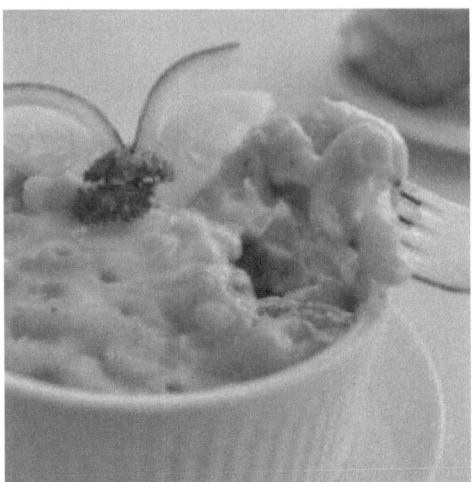

Macaroni and cheese dishes are children's favorites and you can never go wrong with this combination. Add chicken to the duo and you are good to go.

Ingredients

- 2 boiled cups each of macaroni and shredded chicken
- 1 cup each of water and sweetcorn
- 4 ounces butter or margarine
- 2 cups milk
- 3 ounces plain flour
- 1 cup grated cheddar cheese
- ½ teaspoon mustard powder
- Salt and pepper seasoning

Method

1. Preheat oven to 200 degrees C. In a pan over medium heat, melt 1-ounce butter. Add an ounce flour, salt, mustard powder and pepper, mixing thoroughly. Gradually but briskly whisk in the milk and water. Reduce heat and cook while stirring continuously.

2. Remove from heat after sauce thickens. Add macaroni, chicken, ¾ cup cheese and sweetcorn and mix thoroughly. Pour into greased

baking dish and top with remainder of cheese. Bake until golden brown then serve hot.

Note

For variety, you can substitute chicken with pork chops but make sure to remove all fat first.

Recipe 34: Confetti Spaghetti Salad

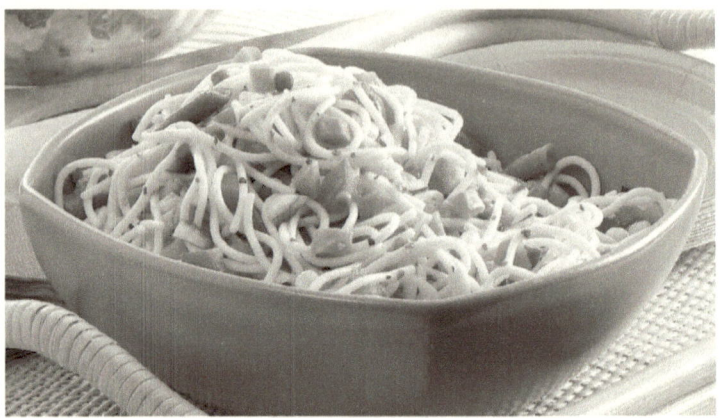

This is an appetizing comfort dish with a colorful appeal. It is very easy to prepare and also has few and easily obtainable ingredients

Ingredients

- 1 7 ounces packet spaghetti, uncooked and broken into thirds
- 2 cups frozen mixed vegetables
- ¼ cup onion, chopped
- ¾ cup chopped tomato
- ½ cup salad dressing

Method

1. Boil spaghetti in a large saucepan with a lot of water and add frozen vegetables in last five minutes. Drain and allow to cool.

2. In a medium sized bowl, toss all ingredients gently and thoroughly mixed. Cover salad and refrigerate for 45 minutes to an hour before serving.

Did you know?

There are more than 600 pasta shapes produced worldwide and most are found in particular regions of the world and not in the others.

Recipe 35: Beef and Curry Pasta

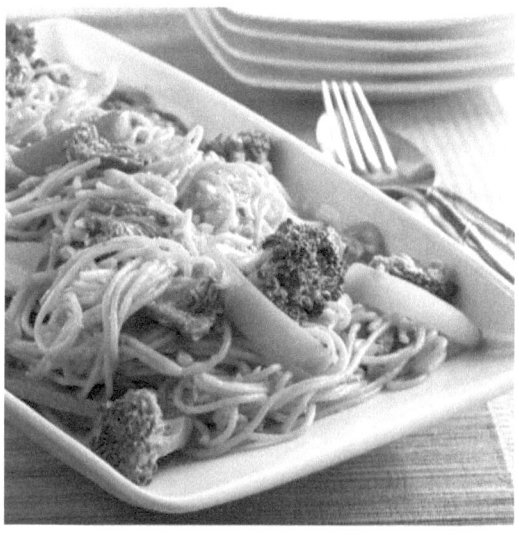

This is an appetizing, scrumptious and filling dish which will keep you going for hours. The curry is just enough to make you feel all fuzzy inside.

Ingredients

- 1-pound macaroni
- 4 teaspoons curry paste
- 1 cup milk
- 3 tablespoons fish sauce
- 2 pounds steak or chuck roast in sizable pieces
- 8 ounces mushrooms
- Medium onion and carrot both sliced thinly
- 10 ounces cauliflower florets
- 2 teaspoons salt
- ½ teaspoon pepper
- 12 ounces trimmed fresh green beans

Method

1. Whisk the paste, milk and sauce in the slow cooker. Add remaining ingredients except beans and stir to ensure sauce coats everything. Add beans but do not mix.

2. Cook on low heat for 8 hours, in the last 30 minutes, stir in beans at ten-minute intervals. Cook pasta according to packet instructions in the last 15 minutes before curry is done. Put drained pasta on a serving dish and top with curry.

Did you know?

Mushrooms are some of the oldest living vegetables and have been used as medicine for thousands of years.

Recipe 36: Tandoori Chicken

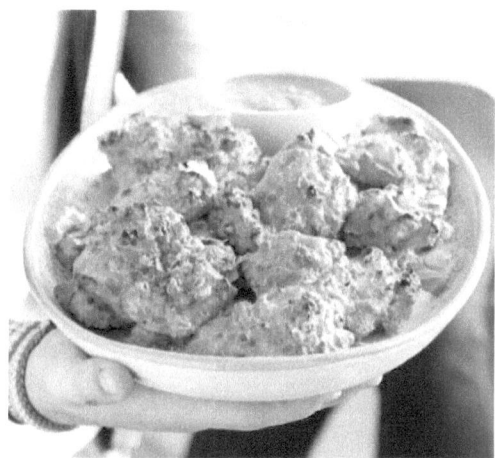

A dish that will make you forget the here and the now as it takes you back to the old days when the stress of adult life fell on someone's shoulders.

Ingredients

- 1 cup, thick and plain yogurt
- 1 garlic clove, crushed
- Peeled and grated ginger piece
- 1 tablespoon each of lemon juice and olive oil
- 1 teaspoon each of masala and ground coriander
- ½ teaspoon each of chili powder and turmeric
- 6 chicken thigh fillets, trimmed
- Cooked rice

Method

1. Mix well yogurt, ginger, garlic, lemon juice, spices, oil and salt in a large bowl. Double slit the top of each thigh without cutting all the way through. Put chicken in mixture making sure to coat well. Refrigerate for 3½ hours.

2. Preheat oven to 220 degrees C towards the end of the refrigeration time. Place chicken in a lined dish and roast until thoroughly cooked. Serve with the rice.

Recipe 37: Spiced Salmon with Chili Sauce

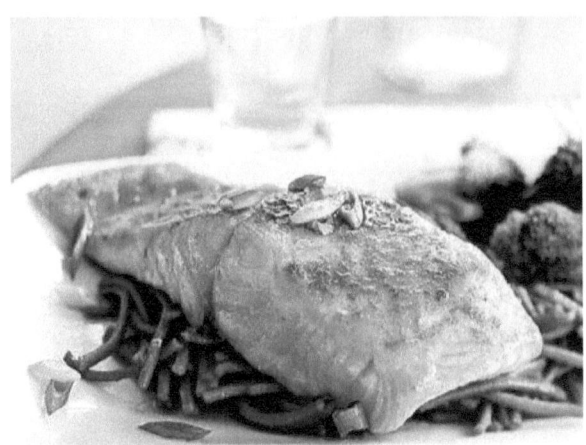

With only 325 calories per serving, this dish is a sure way of enjoying good food while losing weight. The dish gives you comfort without guilt.

Ingredients

- 4 x 6 ounces salmon fillets
- 2 teaspoon chili sauce
- 1 teaspoon honey
- ¼ teaspoon each of ground red pepper, ground turmeric and salt
- ⅛ teaspoon garlic powder

Method

1. Preheat cooking spray coated broiler. Combine all ingredients except the fish in a bowl and stir with a fork.

2. Rub mixture evenly over fish. Place fillets on broiler, skin-side down. Broil for 8-10 minutes.

Did you know?

The spices in this dish will help speed up the metabolic process and therefore help you shed any weight you might want to or help you maintain your weight even as you enjoy comfort food.

Recipe 38: Slow Cooked Stuffed Gammon

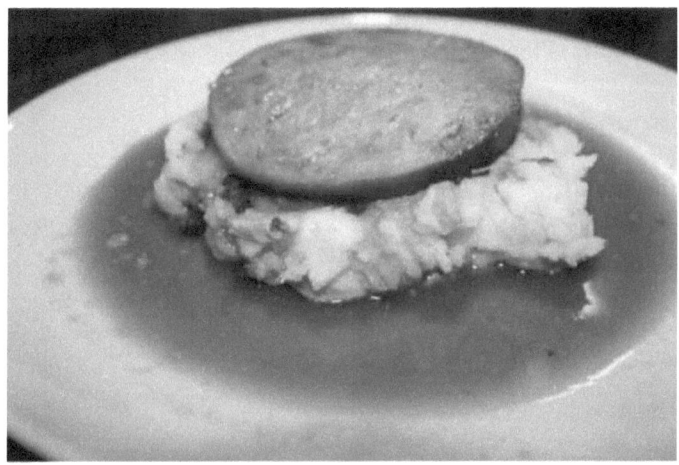

The main ingredient in this dish is beef, and beef is one of the greatest sources of protein. Beef will help you get to the desired amount of proteins per day and because it has no carbs, you can be sure you keep on track of your desired weight loss endeavor.

Ingredients

- 4 pounds boneless gammon
- 1 1 tablespoon oil
- 2 tablespoons curry paste
- 1 cup cooked couscous
- 1 cup dried apples, chopped
- 1 cup dried cranberries
- ½ cup each of pine nuts and maple syrup
- 2 tablespoons vegetable stock
- 2 tablespoon course mustard
- Salt and pepper

Method

1. Grease the crock pot. Make a big hole in the center of the gammon using a flat, sharp knife. Heat oil in a saucepan and add curry, couscous, apples, cranberries and nuts. Season well, remove from the pan and leave to cool.

2. Stuff into gammon and secure with kitchen string. Place in crock pot. Close and cook for 6 hours on low heat. In a bowl, combine syrup, stock and mustard. Pour over gammon and cook again for two hours. Place in oven to brown.

Did you know?

Berries are good for your memory. They contain flavonoids which can improve memory, learning and general cognitive function including reasoning, decision making and verbal comprehension.

Recipe 39: Potato and Pork Bake

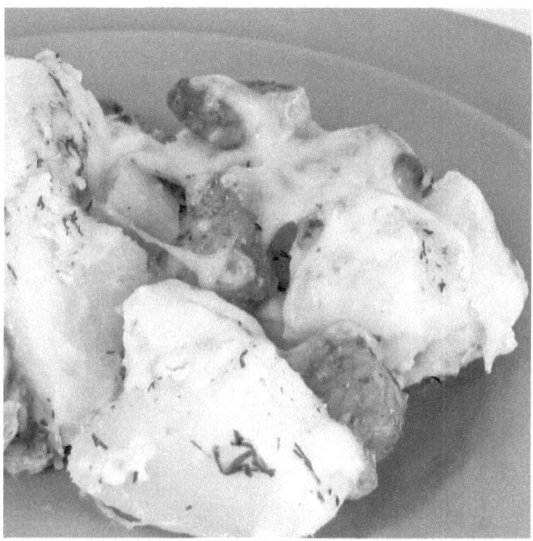

Potatoes are the ultimate comfort food as they always take you back many years. The starchy make up gives the potato its filling quality.

Ingredients

- 8 potatoes cubed
- 8 thick cut pork chops
- 1 onion chopped
- 250 ml vegetable stock

Method

1. Preheat oven to 200 degrees C. Place the potatoes in a baking tray. Arrange the chops over the potatoes.

2. Fry onion until slightly browned and mix with stock. Pour this over the meat and potatoes. Bake for 30 to 40 minutes.

Did You Know?

The now so common vegetable was at some time in its history considered inedible and even poisonous.

Recipe 40: Summer Cabbage Soup with Sausages

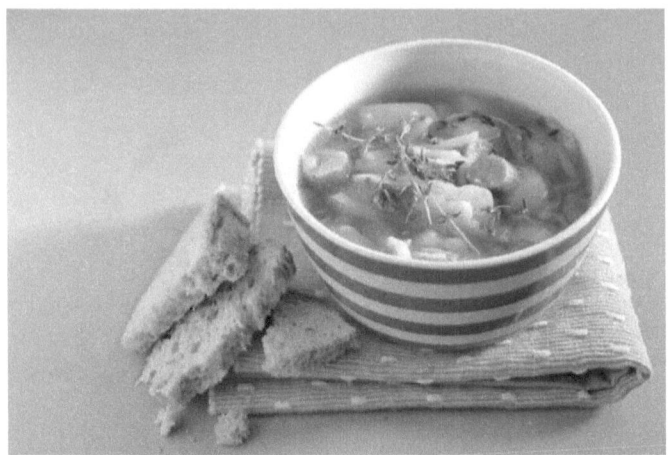

The sausage and cabbage combination in this dish makes the dish highly feeling and ensures loss of weight through keeping you full for longer.

Ingredients

- 4 tablespoons oil
- 1 chopped onion
- 1 sprig thyme
- 8 ounces pork sausages, cooked and sliced
- 1 cabbage, shredded
- 4 medium potatoes, cubed
- 6 cups vegetable stock
- Pepper to taste

Method

1. Heat the oil in a saucepan. Fry the onions in oil until soft. Add the remaining ingredients. Cover and cook for 10-15 minutes. Season well and serve.

Did you know?

Potatoes contain nutrients like vitamin C, B and potassium which are good for relieving inflammation of the intestines and the digestive system.

Recipe 41: Teriyaki Fried Rice with Chicken

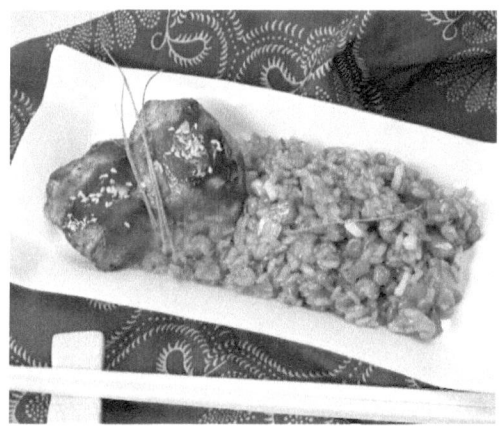

Any meal with chicken is guilt-free comfort food. Chicken is high in protein and therefore low in calories. This allows you to enjoy your food without worrying about weight gain.

Ingredients

- 5 ounces chicken breasts
- 1½ tablespoon vegetable oil
- 2 onions, chopped
- Small carrot, julienned
- Small beaten egg
- 2½ cups cold cooked rice
- 2 tablespoons roasted garlic teriyaki marinade and sauce
- 1 teaspoon chili paste
- 1 tablespoon soy sauce

Method

1. Cut chicken into thin strips. Heat oil in large skillet over high heat. Place chicken, onions, carrot and chili sauce into skillet and stir-fry until chicken is cooked.

2. Gently stir in the egg until firm then add rice and cook until thoroughly heated. Add Teriyaki and soy sauce before you remove from heat and mix well.

Fun fact

Over 50 billion chickens are reared annually for their meat and eggs, making chickens the most populous bird in the world.

Recipe 42: Sea Bass with Orange and Honey

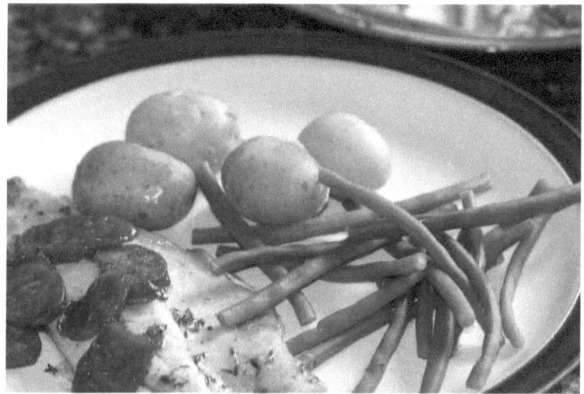

Honey is a naturally warming delicacy whose inclusion here gives the dish a comforting quality that is unmatched.

Ingredients

- 2 large sea-bass fillets
- Zest and juice ½ orange
- 2 teaspoon each honey and mustard
- 2 tablespoon olive oil
- 9 ounces ready-to-eat lentils
- 3 ounces watercress
- Small bunch each parsley and dill, chopped

Method

1. Heat oven to 200^0C. Place fillets skin-down on individual foils. Mix honey, zest, mustard, ½ oil and some seasoning; drizzle mixture over fillets. Pull foil sides up and twist edges.

2. Place foils on baking tray and bake for 10-12 minutes. Warm lentils and mix with remaining ingredients. Divide into 2 plates, place fish on top and drizzle any left juices and serve.

Recipe 43: Slow Cooker Breakfast Casserole

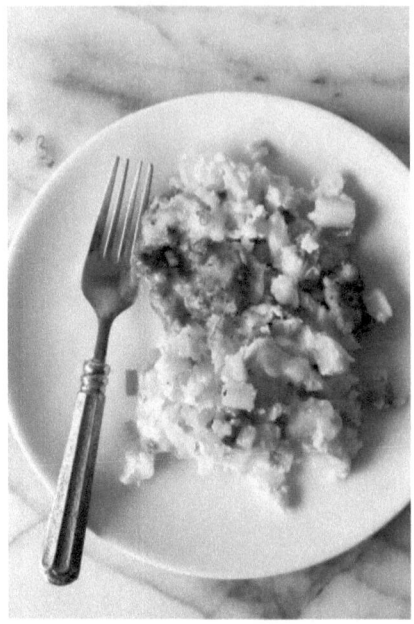

This dish is a filling breakfast dish that has essential nutrients to keep you going and fulfilled for several hours.

Ingredients

- ½ pound ground sausage, browned and drained
- 6 large eggs
- ½ cup milk
- 1-pound frozen hash-browns
- ½ cup salsa
- ½ cup grated cheddar cheese
- ½ pound potatoes
- Salt and pepper to taste

Method

1. Spray non-stick cooking spray into the crock pot. Thoroughly mix together beaten eggs, milk and the salt and pepper before pouring into the cooker.

2. Add the remaining ingredients and stir a little. Cook on low heat for six hours until mixture sets at the center.

Did you know?

Eggs are good for alertness. The protein in egg is an essential component of neurotransmitters like dopamine and norepinephrine which help communication between brain cells.

Recipe 44: Slow Cooker Jambalaya

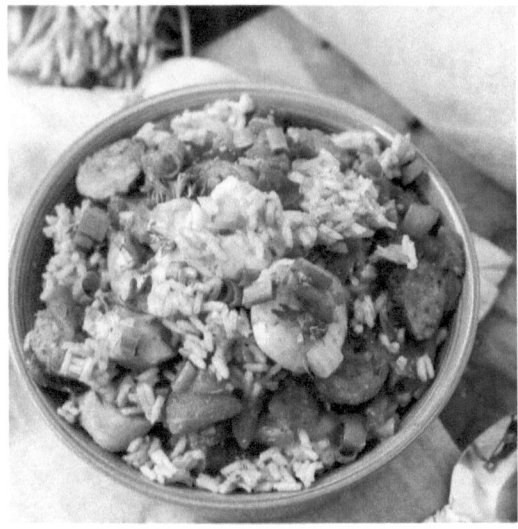

This dish is rich in spices and spices are known for greatly aiding weight loss. Spices are known to speed up metabolism which in turn helps you lose weight faster.

Ingredients

- 1 cup chopped onion
- 1 cup chopped green pepper
- 1 cup chopped celery
- 2 garlic cloves, minced
- 1 28 ounces can un-drained diced tomatoes
- ¾ pound cooked prawns
- 2 cups turkey sausage or smoked sausage
- ¼ teaspoon each of hot sauce and pepper
- ½ teaspoon each of salt and dried thyme
- 1 tablespoon dried parsley

Method

1. Add all ingredients except prawns and stir well. Cook on high for 3-4 hours. Add prawns to crock pot for the last 15 minutes of cooking time.

Did you know?

Tomato is not a vegetable but a fruit and that it helps keep you focused. It also has the potential of positive mood creation and overall clarity.

Recipe 45: Spaghetti Bolognaise

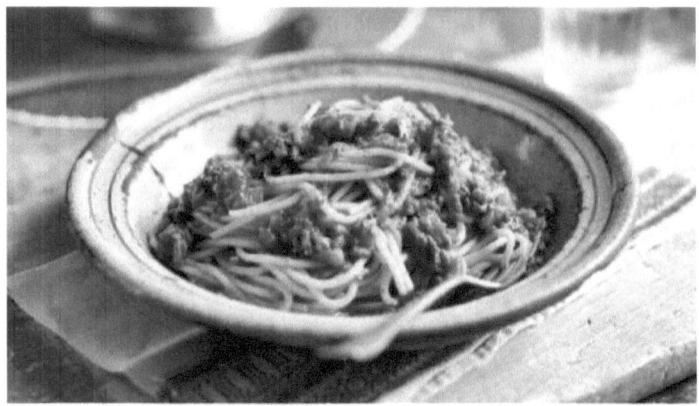

This is a tasty comfort and filling dish which will remind you of those by-gone days and keep you going for hours.

Ingredients

- 1 tablespoon olive oil
- 200 g beef mince
- 1 small onion, sliced
- A chopped garlic clove
- 50 g grated carrots
- 400g tin chopped tomatoes
- 200ml beef stock
- 200 g spaghetti
- Salt and pepper

Method

1. Heat a little oil and fry mince over low heat until browned. Remove from pan and add remaining oil, fry onions until softened. Add garlic and seasoning then fry for two more minutes.

2. Add carrot, mince and tomatoes, stir well to mix. Stir in stock and allow to simmer gently. Cook pasta according to packet instructions. When pasta is cooked, drain and add to sauce and mix well.

Did you know?

In some cultures, garlic is not only considered good for health but even for keeping evil spirits at bay.

Recipe 46: Beef and Vegetable Parmesan

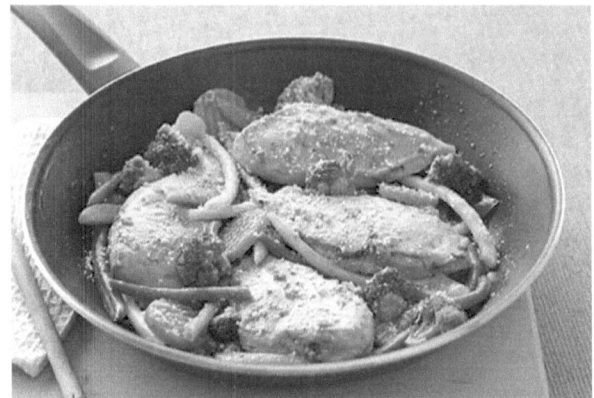

This tasty comfort dish has easily available ingredients has a total of only between 2225 and 2300kj per serving. It has net carbs of 7g per serving.

Ingredients

- 1-pound boneless beef sirloin
- 4 cups broccoli florets
- 2 cups cauliflower florets
- 5 tablespoons shredded parmesan cheese
- 2-3 tablespoons olive oil
- Salt and freshly ground pepper

Method

1. Cut beef into sizable pieces. Sprinkle seasoning. Put a layer of the vegetables on the crock pot. Place the meat on top and add the remaining vegetables on the sides and on top of the meat.

2. Add about 50 milliliters of water. Cook on medium heat for 3-4 hours. Sprinkle the cheese on top before serving.

Did you know?

Olive oil is rich in the anti-oxidant hydroxytyrosol. Anti-oxidants help protect the body against the damage caused by free radicals. The fresher the olive oil, the better the taste and the flavor.

Recipe 47: Fried Green Tomatoes

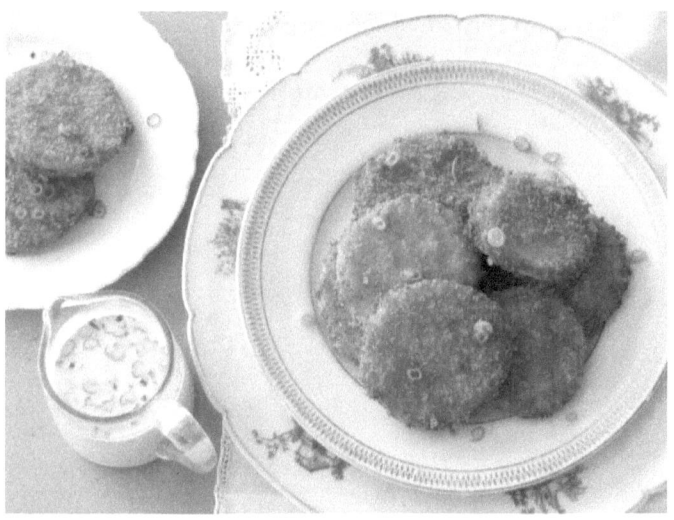

Comfort eating with an easy cooking method and few ingredients is difficult to resist and this is one such a dish with the additional pleasure of great taste.

Ingredients

- 1 lightly beaten egg
- ½ cup each of cornmeal mix, flour and buttermilk
- salt and pepper
- 2 large green tomatoes sliced 5mm thick
- 1 cup vegetable oil

Method

1. Whisk buttermilk and egg. Mix together cornmeal, ½ the flour and salt and pepper in a mixing bowl. Coat tomatoes in remaining flour before dipping into egg and buttermilk mixture then coat with cornmeal mixture.

2. Heat oil in skillet over high heat and reduce heat when oil begins smoking. Gently place coated tomatoes in batches and cook until golden. Remove from oil and drain. Season before serving.

Note

Buttermilk is called for in many recipes even though it is not as widely used as it used to be. You can therefore use substitutes for the milk and this won't change the taste if you use a substitute with an acid to maintain the characteristic flavor.

Recipe 48: Mushroom and Cabbage Stroganoff

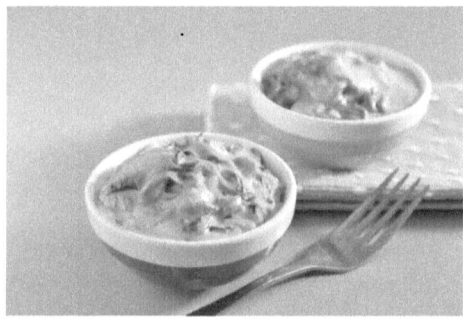

It is not every time that you get comfort food that has the potential to aid in weight loss. The protein in this dish is obtained from the mushrooms and keeps you full for a long time and prevents hunger pangs.

Ingredients

- 4 tablespoons oil
- 1 large onion, chopped
- 2 tablespoons paprika
- 4 pounds sliced mushrooms
- 1 white and 1 red cabbages, shredded
- 3½ cups vegetable stock
- 1-pound double cream
- Salt and pepper

Method

1. Heat oil in a large frying pan, Add onions and fry until soft. Add paprika, cabbage and mushrooms and cook for 3 minutes.

2. Add stock and simmer covered, for 8 minutes. Add the cream and season well then cook for a further 4 minutes before serving.

Did you know?

Cabbage is a cruciferous vegetable a type of vegetables linked to significant reduction in risk of variant cancers. In addition, cabbage can stop running tummies and improve appetite.

Recipe 49: Beef and Portobello Stroganoff

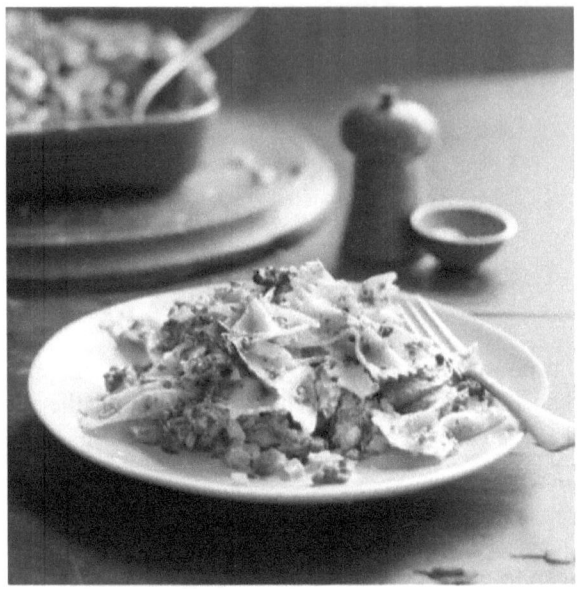

Comfort food with many health benefits from nutrient rich mushrooms. Most mushroom types are even good for your bladder because of the presence of the mineral selenium.

Ingredients

- 4 tablespoons oil
- 1 large onion, chopped
- 2 tablespoons paprika
- 4 pounds sliced Portobello mushrooms
- 2 pounds cubed beef
- 3½ cups vegetable stock
- 1-pound double cream
- Salt and pepper

Method

1. Heat oil in a large frying pan and fry beef until tender and browned. Add onions and fry until soft. Add paprika and mushrooms and cook for 5 minutes.

2. Add stock and simmer covered, for 12 minutes. Add the cream and season well then cook for a further 6 minutes before serving.

Note

There are poisonous varieties of mushrooms and most mushrooms are also easily affected by the surrounding plants and trees so be careful about the mushrooms if they are not store bought.

Recipe 50: Chili Con Carne

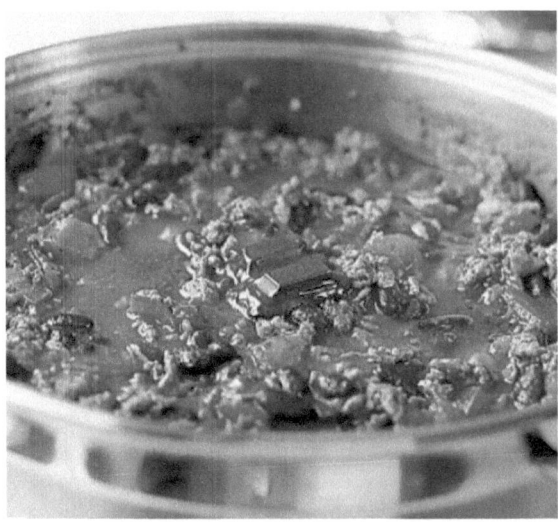

This dish gives you a lot of freedom to maneuver as you can include and drop off some ingredients which are not main, and still come out with a good dish.

Ingredients

- 1-pound minced beef
- 1 medium sized onion, chopped
- 3 finely chopped garlic cloves
- ½ tablespoon each of ground cumin and dried oregano
- 1 tablespoon ground chili peppers
- Salt and pepper seasoning
- 1 cup each of beef broth, cooked kidney beans and tomato puree
- 1 large tomato, chopped
- Cheddar cheese, grated
- Chopped onion

Method

1. Sauté ground beef, onion and garlic in a saucepan until meat changes color. Drain off and discard fat. Add all ingredients except beans then allow to simmer for 3-4 hours, pot uncovered.

2. In last 30 minutes of cooking, add beans, mix thoroughly and continue to simmer. Taste and adjust seasoning if desired.

Did You Know?

You would enjoy the chili better if you allow the flavors to mingle overnight, refrigerated. So, if possible, prepare dish a day before then reheat when you are ready to serve.

Recipe 51: Baked Sweet Potatoes with Sour Cream

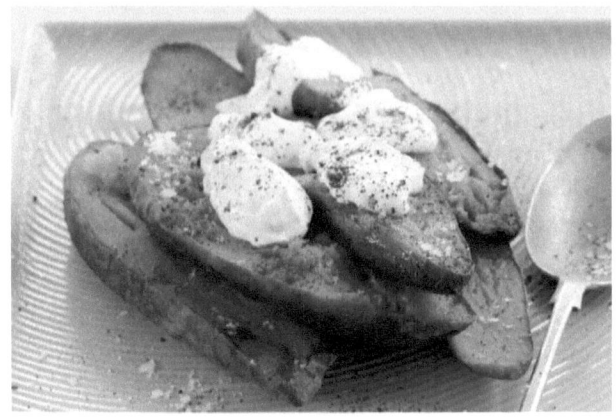

This is a fairly easy dish to make and you can have it ready in just over an hour both prep and cooking time.

Serves 2

Ingredients

- 2 medium sized sweet potatoes, scrubbed
- ¼ cup sour cream
- ½ tablespoon maple syrup

Method

1. Preheat oven to 220 degrees C. Pierce potatoes with a fork and bake on lined baking tray for 50 minutes. Remove from oven and slit potatoes open making sure not to reach the opposite side.

2. Push ends to create an opening. Mix sour cream and maple syrup in a bowl and put a portion in the potato opening. Serve.

Note

Potatoes contain Vitamin C and Vitamin B6. With 132calories for every 100-g potato, they are diet friendly and appetite satisfying at the same time.

Final Words

I would like to thank you for downloading my book and I hope I have been able to help you and educate you about something new.

If you have enjoyed this book and would like to share your positive thoughts, could you please take 30 seconds of your time to go back and give me a review on my Amazon book page!

I greatly appreciate seeing these reviews because it helps me share my hard work!

Again, thank you and I wish you all the best with your cooking journey!

Last Chance to Get YOUR Bonus!

FOR A LIMITED TIME ONLY – Get Olivia's best-selling book *"The #1 Cookbook: Over 170+ of the Most Popular Recipes Across 7 Different Cuisines!"* absolutely FREE!

Readers have absolutely loved this book because of the wide variety of recipes. It is highly recommended you check these recipes out and see what you can add to your home menu!

Once again, as a big thank-you for downloading this book, I'd like to offer it to you *100% FREE for a LIMITED TIME ONLY!*

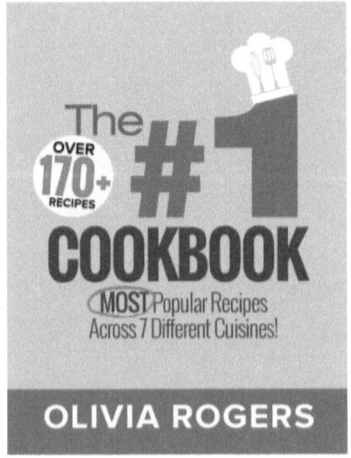

Get your free copy at:

TheMenuAtHome.com/Bonus

Disclaimer

This book and related site provides recipe and food advice in an informative and educational manner only, with information that is general in nature and that is not specific to you, the reader. The contents of this book and related site are intended to assist you and other readers in your personal efforts. Consult your physician or nutritionist regarding the applicability of any information provided in our information to you.

Nothing in this book should be construed as personal advice or diagnosis, and must not be used in this manner. The information provided about conditions is general in nature. This information does not cover all possible uses, actions, precautions, side-effects, or interactions of medicines, or medical procedures. The information in this site should not be considered as complete and does not cover all diseases, ailments, physical conditions, or their treatment.

No Warranties: The authors and publishers don't guarantee or warrant the quality, accuracy, completeness, timeliness, appropriateness or suitability of the information in this book, or of any product or services referenced by this site.

The information in this site is provided on an "as is" basis and the authors and publishers make no representations or warranties of any kind with respect to this information. This site may contain inaccuracies, typographical errors, or other errors.

Liability Disclaimer: The publishers, authors, and other parties involved in the creation, production, provision of information, or delivery of this site specifically disclaim any responsibility, and shall not be held liable for any damages, claims, injuries, losses, liabilities, costs, or obligations including any direct, indirect, special, incidental, or consequences damages (collectively known as "Damages") whatsoever and howsoever caused, arising out of, or in connection with the use or misuse of the site and the information contained within it, whether such Damages arise in contract, tort, negligence, equity, statute law, or by way of other legal theory.

www.ingramcontent.com/pod-product-compliance
Lightning Source LLC
Chambersburg PA
CBHW021127080526
44587CB00012B/1168